AF700441

3D JOINT ANATOMY IN DOGS

Main joint pathologies and surgical approaches

Copyright © 2014 Grupo Asís Biomedia, S.L.
Plaza Antonio Beltrán Martínez nº 1, planta 8 - letra I
(Centro empresarial El Trovador)
50002 Zaragoza - Spain

First printing: June 2014

This book has been published originally in Spanish under the title:
Artrología canina en 3D. Principales patologías ortopédicas y abordajes quirúrgicos
© 2014 Grupo Asís Biomedia, S.L.
ISBN Spanish edition: 978-84-942449-2-6

Translation:
Alexandra Stephens

ISBN: 978-84-942775-5-9
D.L.: Z 888-2014

Design, layout and printing:
Servet editorial - Grupo Asís Biomedia, S.L.
www.grupoasis.com
info@grupoasis.com

Servet is the publishing house of Grupo Asís

All rights reserved.

Any form of reproduction, distribution, publication or transformation of this book is only permitted with the authorisation of its copyright holders, apart from the exceptions allowed by law. Contact CEDRO (Spanish Centre of Reproduction Rights, www.cedro.org) if you need to photocopy or scan any part of this book (www.conlicencia.com; 0034 91 702 19 70/0034 93 272 04 47).

Warning:

Veterinary science is constantly evolving, as are pharmacology and the other sciences. Inevitably, it is therefore the responsibility of the veterinary surgeon to determine and verify the dosage, the method of administration, the duration of treatment and any possible contraindications to the treatments given to each individual patient, based on his or her professional experience. Neither the publisher nor the author can be held liable for any damage or harm caused to people, animals or properties resulting from the correct or incorrect application of the information contained in this book.

3D JOINT ANATOMY in dogs

Main joint pathologies and surgical approaches

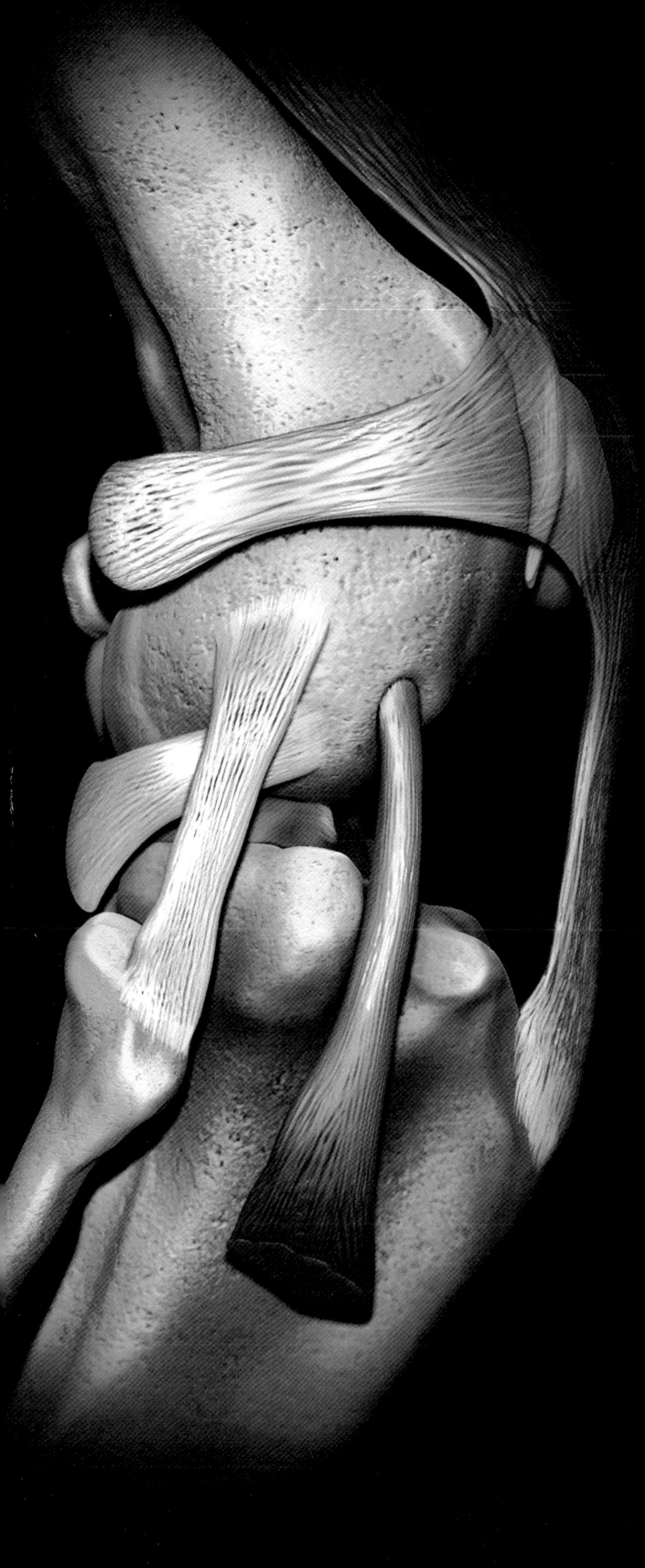

Salvador Climent Peris
Rafael Latorre Reviriego

Roberto Köstlin
José Luis Vérez-Fraguela

Francisco M. Sánchez Margallo
Javier Sánchez Fernández
Diego Celdrán Bonafonte

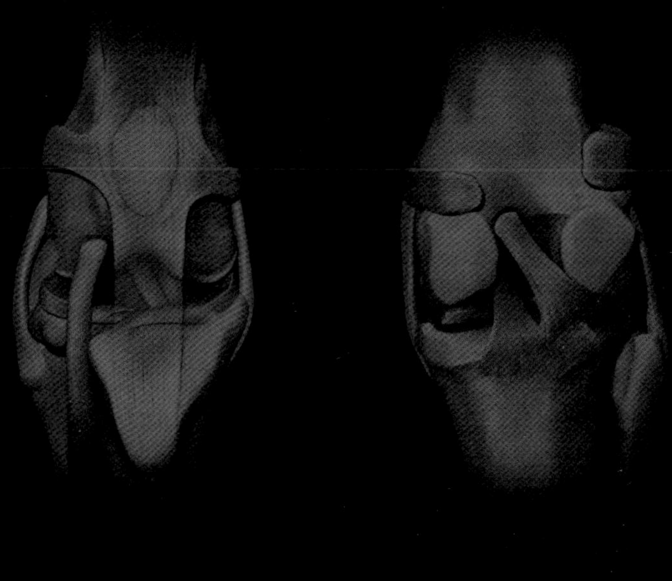

SERVET

AUTHORS

Salvador Climent Peris

Professor Emeritus at the University of Zaragoza since 2012 Graduate in Veterinary Medicine from the University of Zaragoza (Spain), 1969. Professor of Veterinary Anatomy and Embryology since 1982. He has completed terms at the Anatomy Departments of the Faculties of Medicine at the University of Zaragoza, Madrid Complutense University, the Free University of Brussels, the Faculty of Veterinary Medicine in Toulouse, and the Animal Biology Department at the University of Clermont-Ferrand (France). He has been actively involved in the set-up and development of CCMIJU (Minimally Invasive Surgery Centre) in Cáceres, Spain, since 1986, taking part in the design, preparation and selection of appropriate animal models for the specialisation courses in minimally invasive surgical techniques taught at the school.

Rafael Latorre Reviriego

Professor of Veterinary Anatomy, obtaining his Doctorate in Veterinary Medicine in 1990 from the University of Murcia (Spain). He has completed terms at the University of Milan (Italy), Davis (California, USA) Cambridge (UK), Tennessee (USA) and London (UK). A large part of his activity has focused on the clinical anatomy of the locomotion system, in particular significant contributions in the form of anatomy atlases and books, as well as scientific papers published in prestigious journals, mainly relating to image diagnosis of joint conditions. His involvement in the development and teaching of anatomical plastination techniques as a tool for working in clinical anatomy has led him to hold the position of Vice President of the International Society for Plastination.

Roberto Köstlin

Doctor in Veterinary Medicine from the National University of the Northeast, Corrientes (Argentina). Graduate in Veterinary Medicine and training as a tutor at the Ludwig-Maximilians University in Munich (Germany). Diploma from the European College of Veterinary Surgeons (ECVS). Assistant Professor of Surgery at the School of Veterinary Medicine in Hannover (Germany). Assistant Professor of Surgery and Ophthalmology at the Ludwig-Maximilians University in Munich. He has published a number of books and over 100 scientific papers. He has also given countless international conferences around the world.

José Luis Vérez-Fraguela

Graduate and Doctor of Veterinary Medicine and Animal Health from the Faculty of Veterinary Medicine at the University of Extremadura (Spain, UEX). Teaching and research assistant at the Department of Surgery at UEX. Research assistant at the Experimental Surgery Unit at the University Hospital of A Coruña (Spain, CHUAC). Assistant at the Department of Animal Medicine and Health at UEX. Scientific advisor in veterinary orthopaedics for CCMIJU. He has completed terms at Universities in Europe, the USA and Japan. He received the National Research Prize in 1998. He was also granted a European Patent in 2011. He has completed a number of different subsidised research projects, and is a scientific reviewer and member of the scientific and organising committees for a range of different courses, conferences and talks. He has written over 70 publications including books, essays and original papers, and has given countless conferences, talks and courses.

Francisco Miguel Sánchez Margallo

Scientific Director for CCMIJU in Cáceres, Spain. Doctor in Veterinary Medicine from the University of Extremadura (Spain), speaker and director for over 450 national and international training activities, for the practical training of surgeons and other healthcare professionals. He is the author of over 120 publications in scientific journals and over 70 further publications on minimally invasive surgery. With over 10 published books, he has also contributed to over 40 further publications in several languages. He has been involved in over 430 national and international scientific conferences in the field of minimally invasive procedures and surgical technology. He has supervised 12 Doctorates and tutored 4 international Doctorate students, and has directed or taken part in over 70 RDI projects, including European and business projects, as the author of over 10 patents. He is currently a member of several national and international associations relating to health, surgery and health technology, and is a reviewer and member of the editorial committee for different international journals.

Javier Sánchez Fernández

Graduate in Veterinary Medicine from the University of Extremadura (Spain), he is currently writing a thesis in the field of the assessment and optimisation of health training programmes. He has worked as a quality consultant and accredited trainer for many years. He is an assessor for the Commission for Continuous Professional Development for Healthcare in Extremadura and also works with the School of Health Sciences in Extremadura. As a Training Coordinator and Quality Manager for CCMIJU in Cáceres, he has taken part in over 700 training activities and the assessment and supervision of over 7000 healthcare professionals in 17 countries. He is a founder member and Secretary of the Spanish Association for Minimally Invasive Veterinary Medicine and sits on the scientific committees for a number of symposiums and conferences, both national and international.

Diego Celdrán Bonafonte

Graduate in Veterinary Medicine from the University of Extremadura (Spain). Intern at the Departments of Surgery and Pathological Anatomy at the Faculty of Veterinary Medicine in Cáceres (Spain), he has spent most of his professional career in the area of exotic animals. He has completed terms in different national and international institutions as a veterinary surgeon. He was selected by CCMIJU in Cáceres for a pre-Doctorate scholarship to commence his career as a researcher. He currently manages the CCMIJU Animal Modelling Department, while collaborating in the organisation of different training activities in the area of veterinary orthopaedics.

COLLABORATORS

Albarracín López, J. Specialist auxiliary technician. Veterinary Anatomy, University of Murcia (Spain).

Ayala Florenciano, Mª.D. DVM, PhD. Professor of Veterinary Anatomy, University of Murcia (Spain).

Bardet, J.F. DocVet, MS Dip ACVS. Dr. Bardet Surgical Clinic, Neuilly sur Seine, Paris (France).

Boada Villacorta, L. DVM. Ultramar Clinical Veterinary Hospital, Ferrol, Galicia (Spain).

Climent Aroz, M. DVM. Professor of Veterinary Anatomy, University of Zaragoza (Spain).

Domínguez Sarceda, R. DVM. La Castellana Veterinary Clinic, Madrid (Spain).

Gil Cano, F. DVM, PhD. Professor of Veterinary Anatomy, University of Murcia (Spain).

Gómez Uzal, D. DVM. Ultramar Clinical Veterinary Hospital, Ferrol, Galicia (Spain).

Gorostiza, J.F. DVM MS. Surgical Consultation Services, Miami, Florida (USA).

Guerrero, T. Dip ECVS. Surgical Area. St George's University, True Blue (Granada).

Guillén Herrero, S. DVM. Ultramar Clinical Veterinary Hospital, Ferrol, Galicia (Spain).

Henry, R. DVM, PhD. Professor of Veterinary Anatomy, University of Tennessee (USA).

Johnson, K. Professor, MVSc PhD, FACVSc, Dipl ACVS & ECVS. The University of Sydney (Australia).

López Albors, O. DVM, PhD. Professor of Veterinary Anatomy, University of Murcia (Spain).

Luera Carbó, M. DVM PhD. Dr. Luera Veterinary Clinic, Barcelona, Catalonia (Spain). †

Maestre Antequera, J. DU Nurs. Diagnostic Imaging Department, CCMIJU, Cáceres (Spain).

Marti, J.M. LV, Cert SAO, Dip ACVS, Dip ECVS, MRCVS. Veterinary Surgical Specialists, Chesapeake, Virginia (USA).

Martínez Gomariz, F. DVM, PhD. Professor of Veterinary Anatomy, University of Murcia (Spain).

Matis, U. Professor, PhD, Dipl. ECVS. Ludwig-Maximilians-University, Munich (Germany).

Montavon, P. Professor. School of Veterinary Medicine, University of Zurich (Switzerland).

Orenes Hernández, M. Specialist Technician. Veterinary Anatomy, University of Murcia (Spain).

Ramírez Zarzosa, G. DVM, PhD. Professor of Veterinary Anatomy, University of Murcia (Spain).

Ruiz Pérez, M. DVM. Mediterráneo Veterinary Clinic, Madrid (Spain).

Sánchez Collado, C. DVM. Professor of Veterinary Anatomy, University of Murcia (Spain).

Sarriá Cabrera, R. DVM, PhD. Asst in Veterinary Anatomy, University of Murcia (Spain).

Sever Bermejo, R. DVM. Associate Professor, Faculty of Veterinary Medicine, Zaragoza, Aragón (Spain).

Souto Rey, V. DHM. Asst. Doctor of Orthopaedic Surgery at the University Hospital of Ferrol (CHUF), Associate Professor at the Faculty of Podiatry and Nursing in Ferrol, Galicia (Spain).

Suárez Gil, M. 3D technician. Interactive 3D unit , CCMIJU, Cáceres (Spain).

Vázquez Autón, J. DVM, PhD. Professor of Veterinary Anatomy, University of Murcia (Spain).

Villamonte Chevalier, A. Doctorate student in Veterinary Anatomy, University of Murcia (Spain).

FOREWORD

This publication *3D Joint anatomy in dogs - Main joint pathologies and surgical approaches* has three key noteworthy aspects.

Firstly, it is of doubtless clinical value, as it focuses on the six main joints of the dog's body.

Secondly, it is developed in stages, from the clear and precise anatomic context of each and every joint, with a series of real images obtained by CAT and MRI scans, X-rays and even fluoroscopes, and a collection of specially designed three dimensional drawings, together with real plastinated sections to clarify any further doubts that the reader may have. Having provided a clear presentation of the anatomy, the book is complemented with a description of the most common pathologies in canine joints.

All this is required in order to perform the different orthopaedic approaches required to treat these pathologies, brought together in a specific manner in this publication.

The project, which has brought together the work of anatomists, imaging specialists and clinicians from a number of countries, was intended from the outset to be of direct application in orthopaedics and use in daily clinical practice with dogs. The correlation of the CAT and MRI images with real plastinated sections, which facilitate an understanding of the anatomical structures and the consequences of different pathologies, has therefore resulted in an entirely appropriate increase on the part of the authors of the number of images used in relation to the text.

Overall, and considering the importance of diagnostic imaging techniques, this work is not only of interest for clinical professionals but is also relevant to all the recent developments taking place in the field of cell therapy, regarding the regeneration of cartilage and control of inflammation, as the images provided through CAT and MRI scans provide us with a clear and accurate picture of the evolution and monitoring of these aspects.

Given the above, I advise clinical staff to keep a copy of this project among their reference books, for clinical application and consultation purposes.

Prof. Jesús Usón Gargallo

Professor of Surgical Pathology and Surgery
Honorary Chairman of the CCMIJU Foundation

PREFACE

This book has been compiled in an effort to deal with the basic problems faced by veterinary surgeons when handling pathologies in the key joints of the canine limb, presenting the details of each in a logical manner - firstly in depth anatomical information, using all the tools for analysis and representation currently available to us: three-dimensional drawings, animations, simple or three-dimensional CAT and CAT combined with colour angiography, MRI...

This is followed by details of the most common orthopaedic conditions for each joint, in order of prevalence and illustrated with three dimensional drawings, X-rays, surgical images and all details considered relevant to each case.

Where considered appropriate, sections obtained from CAT and MRI scans are compared with transparent plastinated sections of the same area on similar planes, which facilitates the interpretation of the images provided by these diagnostic imaging techniques.

Finally, a variety of key surgical approaches for each region are described step by step, illustrated with photographs taken during anatomical dissection, which we consider to be of great use as they provide a realistic image of the procedure. All the images have been taken from the limbs on the dogs' right, in an attempt to avoid any confusion in interpretation.

We would like to thank Jacob Gragera (Vet and Graduate in Fine Arts) for his work on the completion and processing of the drawings, and the tireless effort of Dr. Tatiana Blasco on coordination tasks, both from the Grupo Asís production department.

The Authors

TABLE OF CONTENTS

2 Hip joint

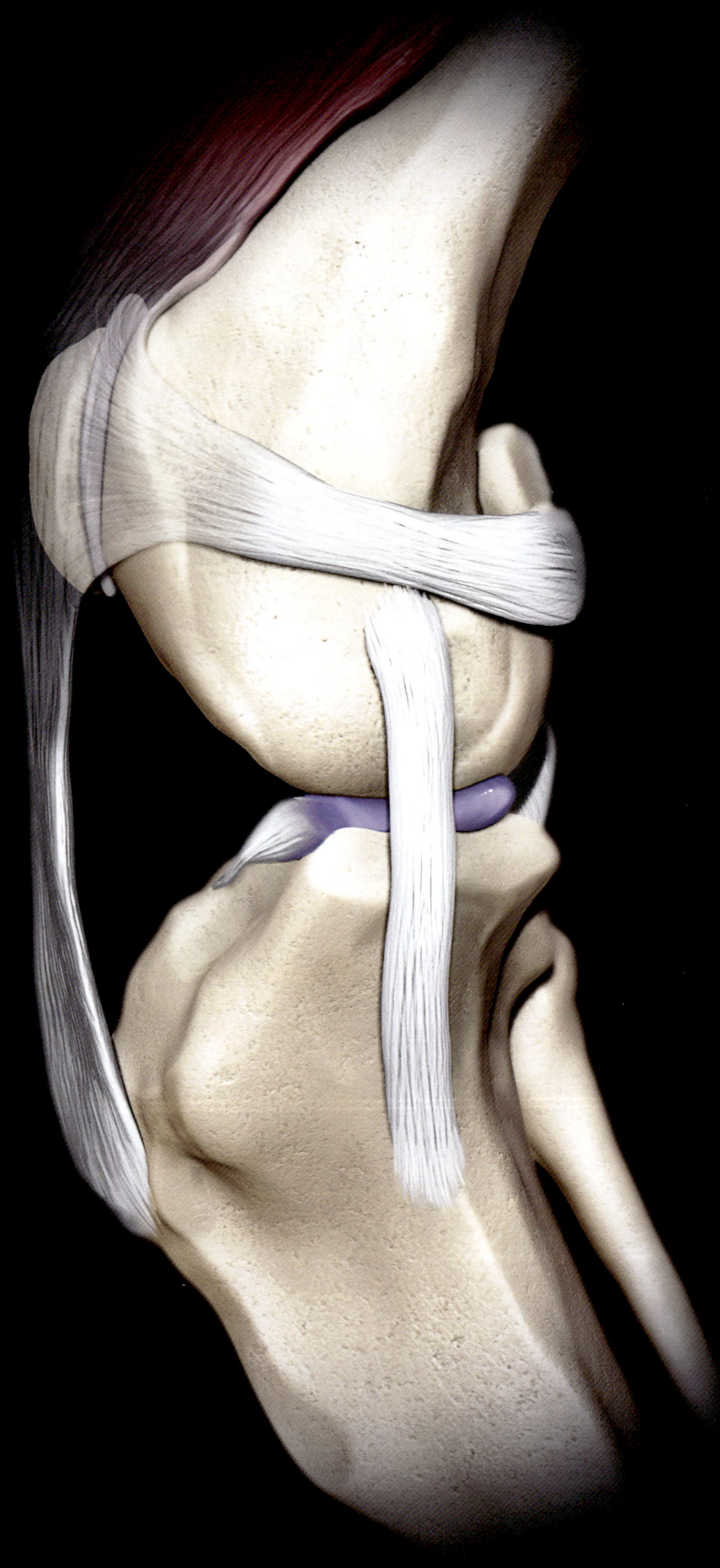

STIFLE JOINT

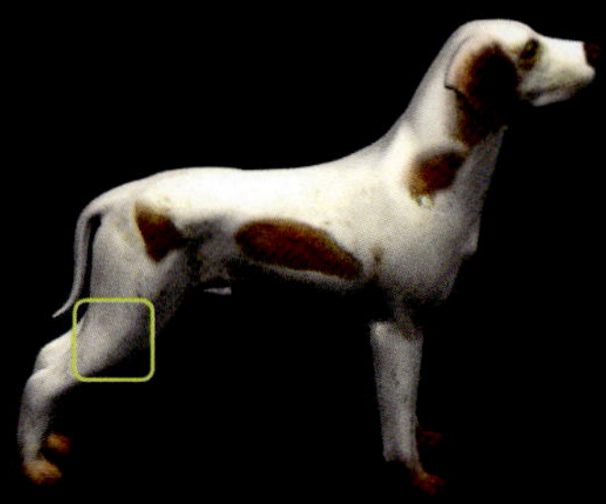

Stifle joint

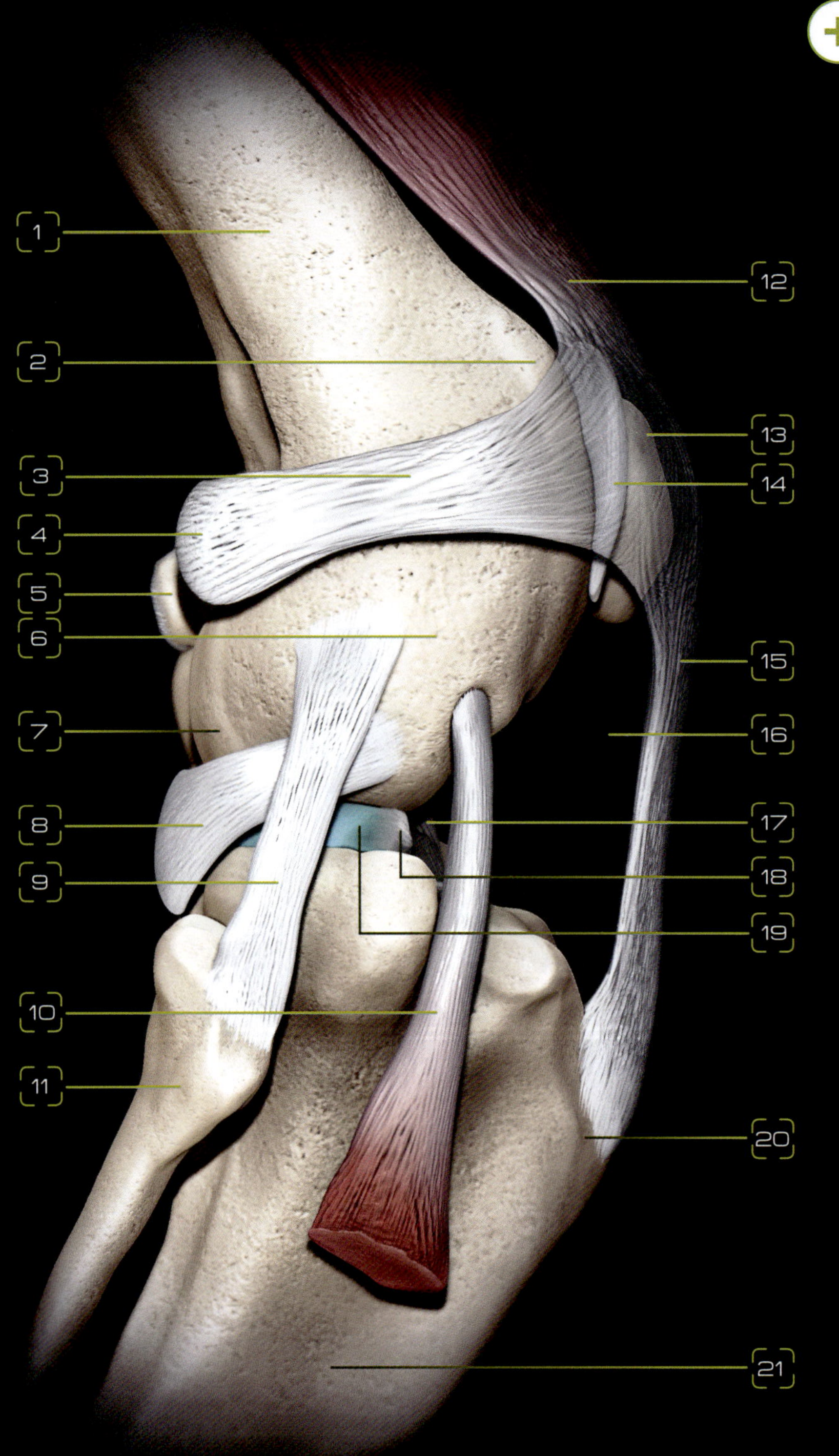

Watch this video on
the electronic version

Full skeleton

LATERAL VIEW

1 Femur
2 Lateral ridge of the trochlea
3 Lateral femoropatellar lig.
4 Lateral gastrocnemius sesamoid bone
5 Medial gastrocnemius sesamoid bone
6 Lateral femoral epicondyle
7 Lateral femoral condyle
8 Tendon of origin of popliteus muscle
9 Lateral collateral lig.
10 Tendon of origin of the long digital extensor muscle
11 Fibula
12 Quadriceps femoris tendon
13 Patella
14 Lateral parapatellar fibrocartilage
15 Patellar lig.
16 Space occupied by infrapatellar fat pad
17 Cranial cruciate lig.
18 Lateral cranial meniscus lig.
19 Lateral meniscus
20 Tibial tuberosity

CAUDAL VIEW

1 Medial femoropatellar lig.
2 Medial gastrocnemius sesamoid bone
3 Medial femoral condyle
4 Medial collateral lig.
5 Medial meniscus
6 Medial tibial condyle
7 Caudal cruciate lig.
8 Caudal lig. of lateral meniscus
9 Lateral femoropatellar lig.
10 Lateral gastrocnemius sesamoid bone
11 Lateral femoral condyle
12 Lateral collateral lig.
13 Meniscofemoral lig.
14 Popliteal muscle tendon
15 Popliteal sesamoid bone

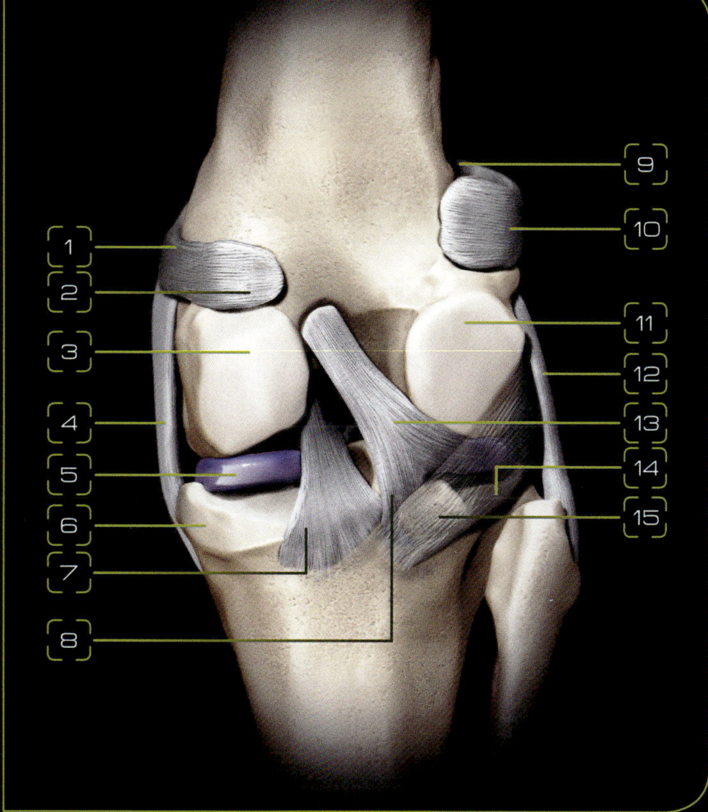

Watch this video on the electronic version

Pelvic limb

MEDIAL VIEW

1 Quadriceps femoris tendon
2 Patella
3 Medial parapatellar fibrocartilage
4 Medial ridge of the trochlea
5 Medial femoral epicondyle
6 Patellar lig.
7 Cranial lig. of medial meniscus
8 Medial femoropatellar lig.
9 Medial femoral condyle
10 Medial meniscus
11 Medial tibial condyle
12 Medial collateral lig.

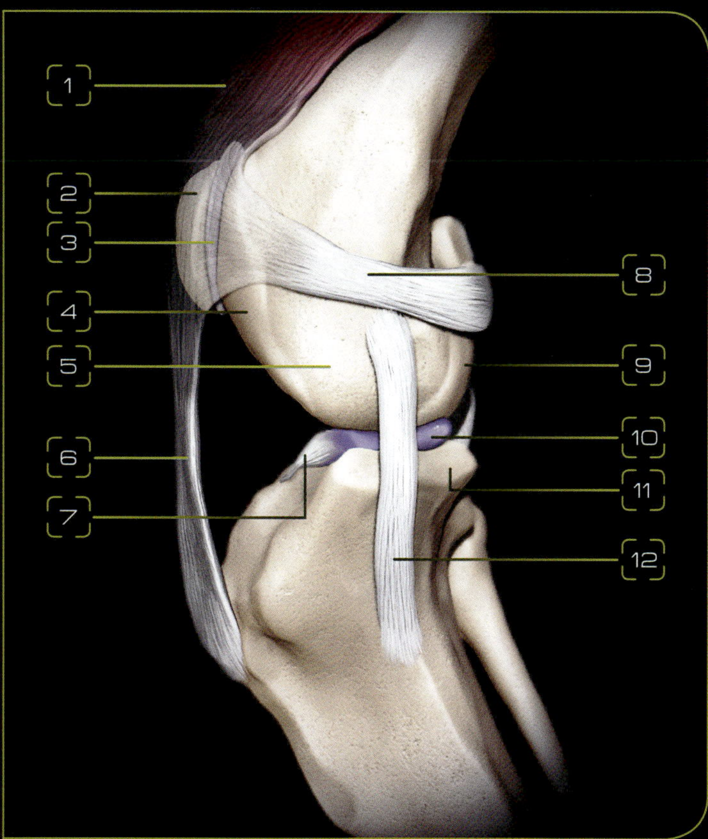

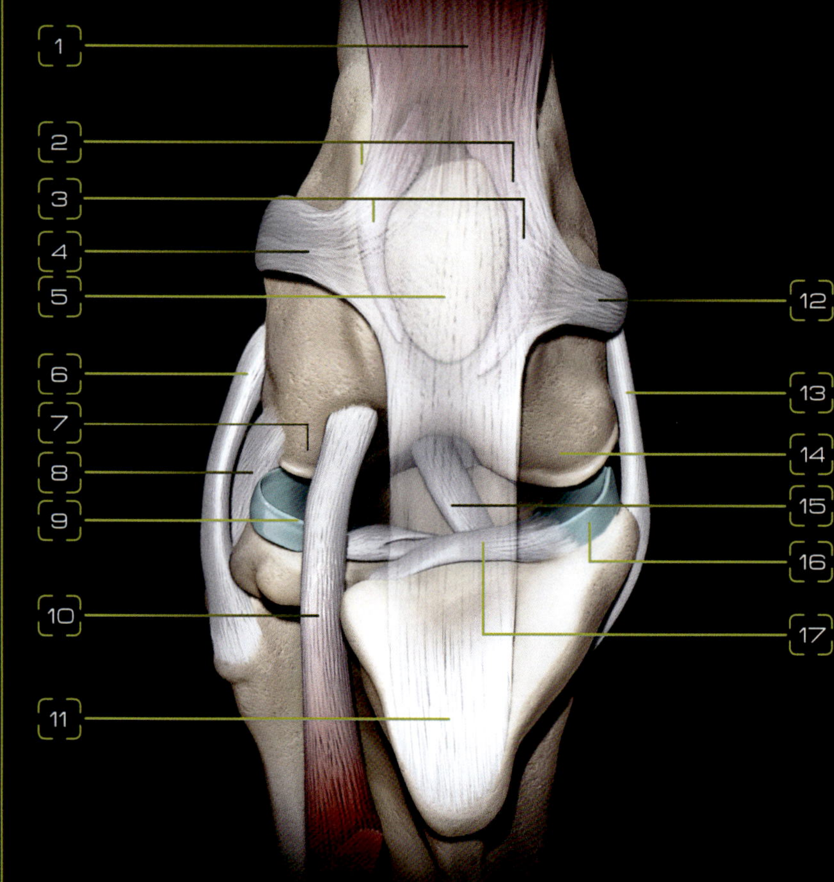

CRANIAL VIEW

1 Quadriceps femoris tendon
2 Femoral trochlea
3 Parapatellar fibrocartilages
4 Lateral femoropatellar lig.
5 Patella
6 Lateral collateral lig.
7 Lateral femoral condyle
8 Popliteal muscle tendon
9 Lateral meniscus
10 Tendon of origin of the long digital extensor muscle
11 Patellar lig.
12 Medial femoropatellar lig.
13 Medial collateral lig.
14 Medial femoral condyle
15 Cranial cruciate lig.
16 Medial meniscus
17 Transverse lig. of stifle joint

Vasculature of the stifle joint

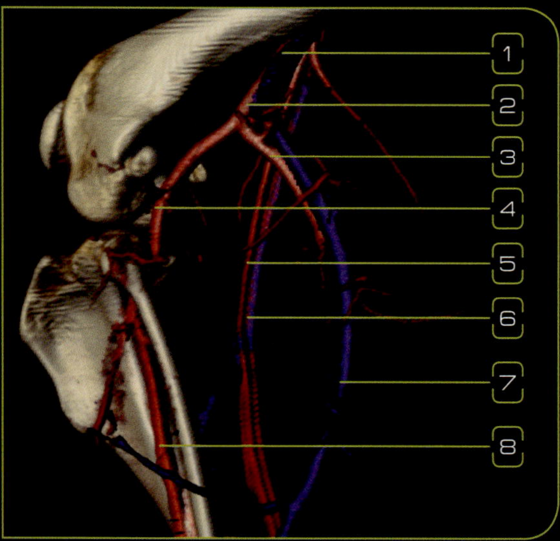

CAUDOLATERAL VIEW

1 Femoral vein
2 Femoral artery
3 Distal caudal femoral artery
4 Popliteal artery
5 Saphenous artery
6 Medial saphenous vein
7 Lateral saphenous vein
8 Cranial tibial artery

Watch this video on the electronic version

CAT - colour angiography

Orthopaedic conditions of the stifle joint

The main orthopaedic conditions of the stifle joint, in order of frequency, are as follows:

01 Rupture of cranial cruciate ligaments

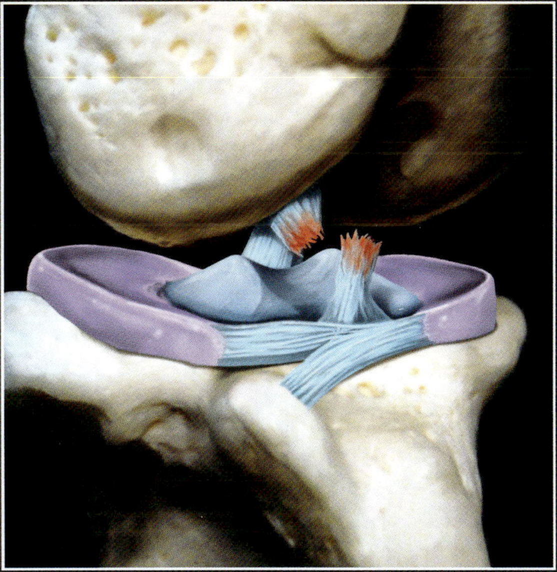

02 Patellar luxation

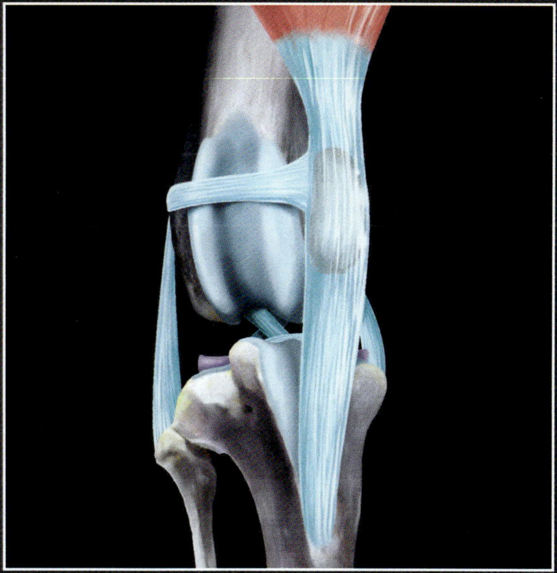

03 Osteochondrosis dissecans

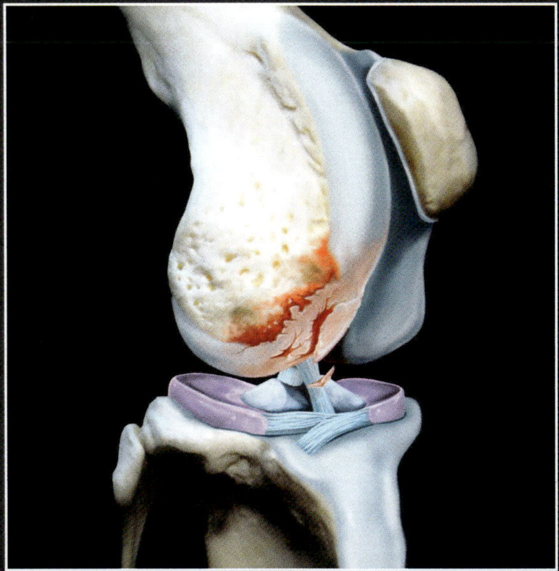

04 Arthritis/osteoarthritis

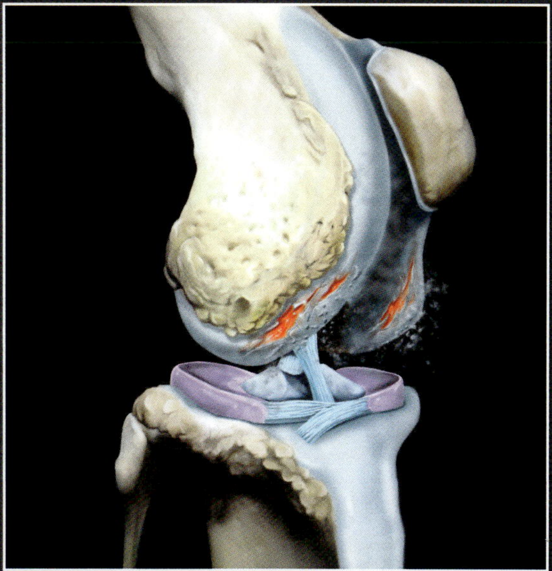

01 Rupture of cruciate ligaments

Clinical signs

- Acute or chronic lameness.
- Joint inflammation.
- Pain on palpation, in particular on hyperextension.
- Positive "drawer test".
- Positive "Finochietto's Jump Test" where there is an injury to the meniscus.
- In chronic cases, hypertrophy of the articular capsule and an increase in synovial fluid.
- Muscular atrophy.
- Osteoarthritic alterations along the trochlear ridge.

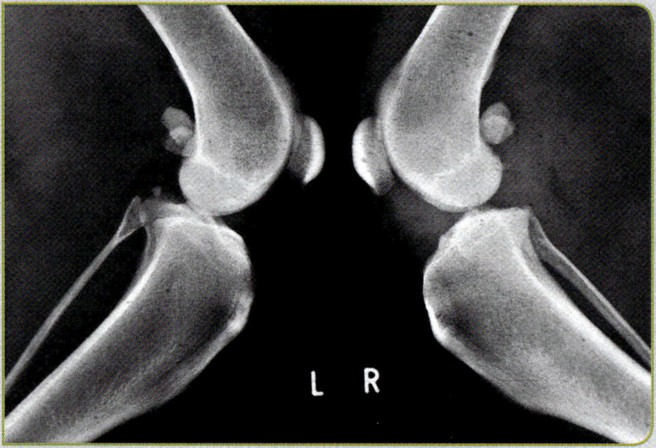

Figure 1. Right stifle joint with an increase in radio density in the articular cavity.

Diagnosis

Diagnosis is based on:

- Clinical history.
- Clinical examination.
- "Drawer test" under local or general anaesthesia.
- X-ray examination (Figs. 1 and 2).

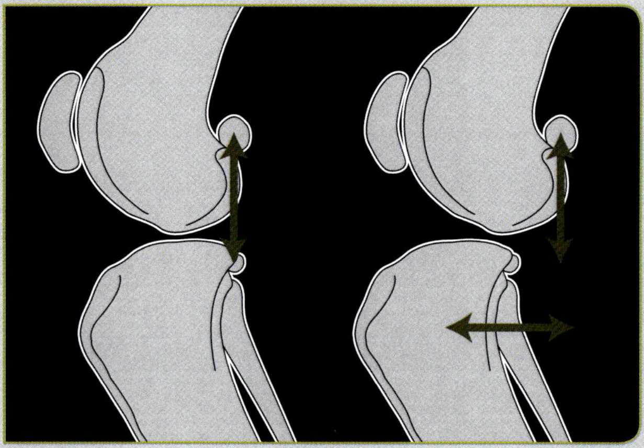

Figure 2. Radiologic sign of positive "drawer test". Cranial displacement of the tibia from the distal femoral epiphysis resulting from a ruptured cranial cruciate ligament.

A diagnosis of ruptured cruciate ligaments can easily be established using the "drawer test". In some larger breeds, and where there is strong muscle contraction, this test may be difficult to perform, and it may be easier to use the "tibial compression test". It is important to remember that this is a less reliable diagnostic test than the first and confirmation of the diagnosis under full muscular relaxation is often required.

To diagnose a rupture of the cranial cruciate ligament the "drawer test" is performed with the stifle joint extended, while for the diagnosis of a rupture of the caudal cruciate ligament the joint remains in flexion. It is important to remember this differentiation as surgery is not necessary to repair caudal cruciate ligaments, as there is full muscular compensation in this case and practically no development of deforming arthropathy.

It is always advisable to examine both limbs, as the condition may be bilateral. One limb may present a recent rupture of the cranial cruciate ligament with aseptic arthritis or injury to the medial meniscus, and the animal may be lame on that side despite suffering a rupture of the cranial cruciate ligament on the opposite limb several weeks previously.

There are a number of different surgical techniques to resolve a rupture of the cranial cruciate ligament (Figs. 3, 4 and 5).

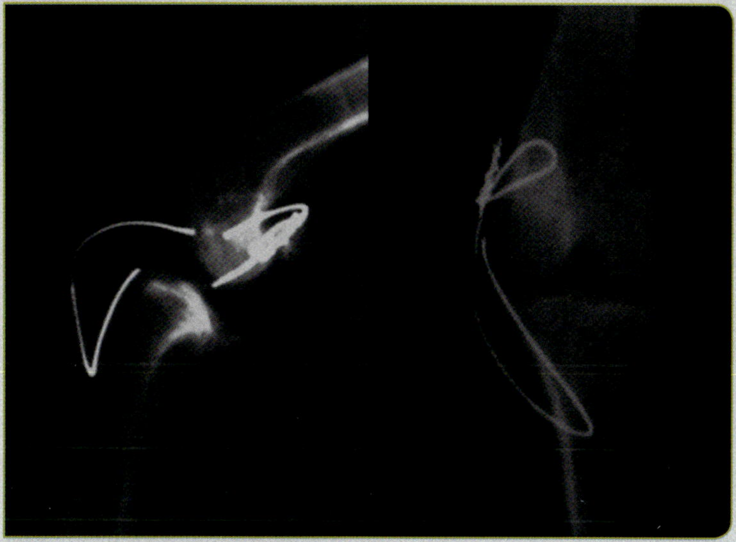

Figure 3. X-ray of a case treated using the Olmstead technique, showing severe signs of osteoarthritis.

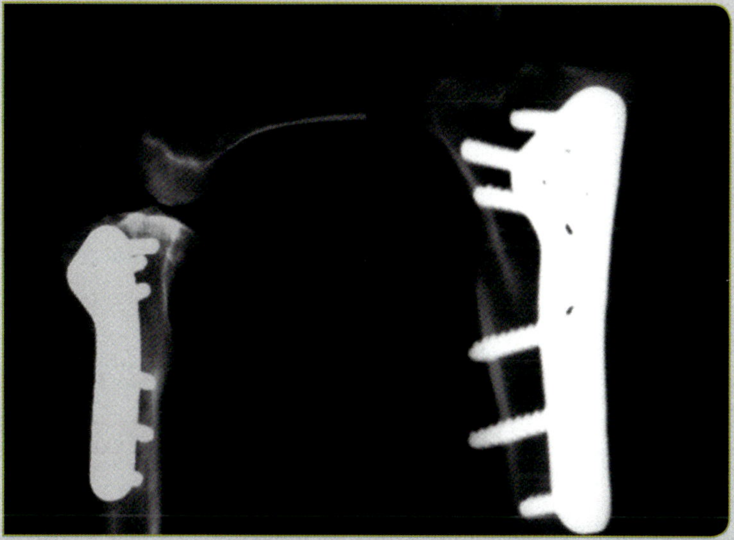

Figure 4. X-ray of a case treated with TPLO (Tibial Plateau Levelling Osteotomy) after several years without signs of osteoarthritis.

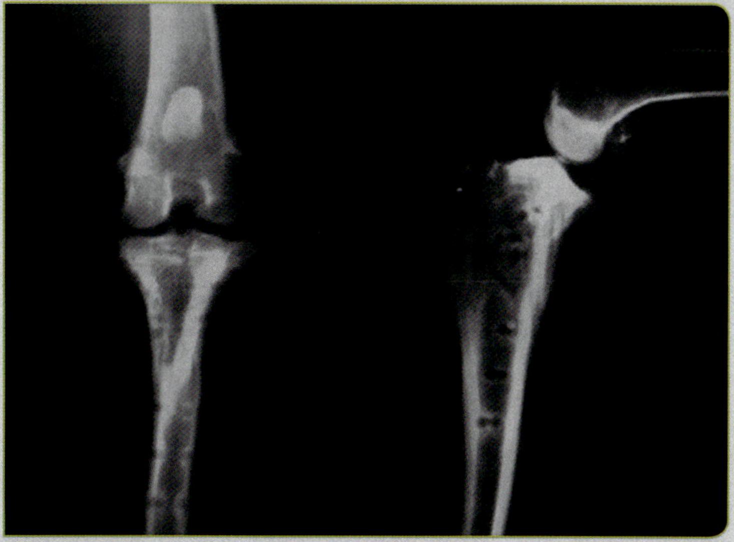

Figure 5. Postoperative X-ray after removal of the TPLO implant shown above, with little sign of osteoarthritis.

02 Patellar luxation

This is a very common orthopaedic condition. It is found particularly in smaller breeds, but also in some large breeds (Samoyed, Eurasier) and in cats.

There are different types of luxation:

- Medial (Fig. 6).
- Lateral.
- Medial and lateral.
- Trauma-induced.

In the case of medial luxation in toy breeds, there are 4 grades (Fig. 7):

- **Grade I:** the patella luxates easily with the stifle extended; upon release it moves only towards the femoral condyles. This is normally a common luxation with intermittent lameness. Tibial rotation is minimal and upon flexing the stifle it remains aligned with no abduction of the tarsus.
- **Grade II:** the patella is often displaced outside the intercondylar articular groove. The limb is used with the stifle joint in flexion. Upon examination under general anaesthesia, the patella can be reduced by lateral rotation of the tibia, and upon release of the tibia it luxates spontaneously. The tibia can be rotated around 30° off the sagittal plane. As the patella is luxated medially, abduction of the tarsus can be observed.
- **Grade III:** the patella is permanently luxated and the tibia can be rotated around 30-60°. The limb can be used, but with the stifle in flexion.
- **Grade IV:** the tibial tuberosity can be rotated around 60-90°. The patella is permanently luxated. The limb generally cannot be used and it is difficult to located the patella by palpation. An X-ray of the stifle in flexion (skyline) shows the depth of the femoral trochlear groove (Figs. 8 and 9).

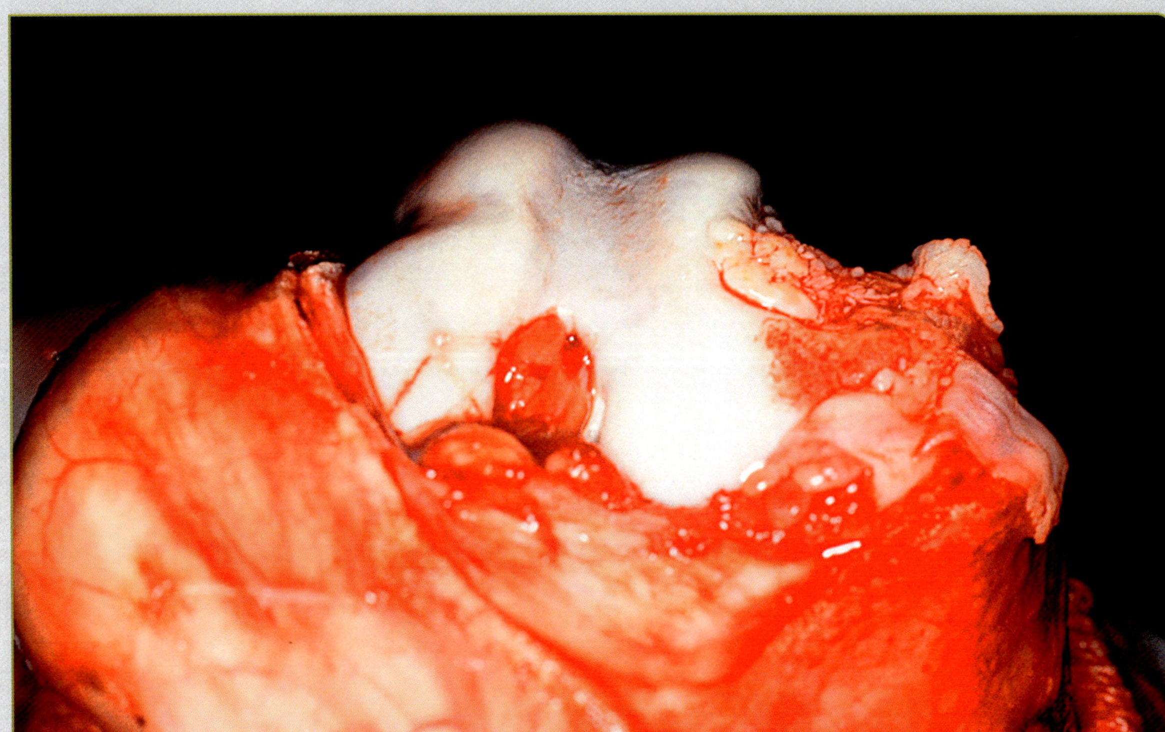

Figure 6. Surgical image of a case of patellar luxation. The medial displacement of the patella causes a groove to form over the osteophytes over which the luxated patella moves.

Figure 7. Grades of patellar luxation (adapted from Brinker, Piermattei and Flo's Handbook of Small Animal Orthopaedics and Fracture Repair).

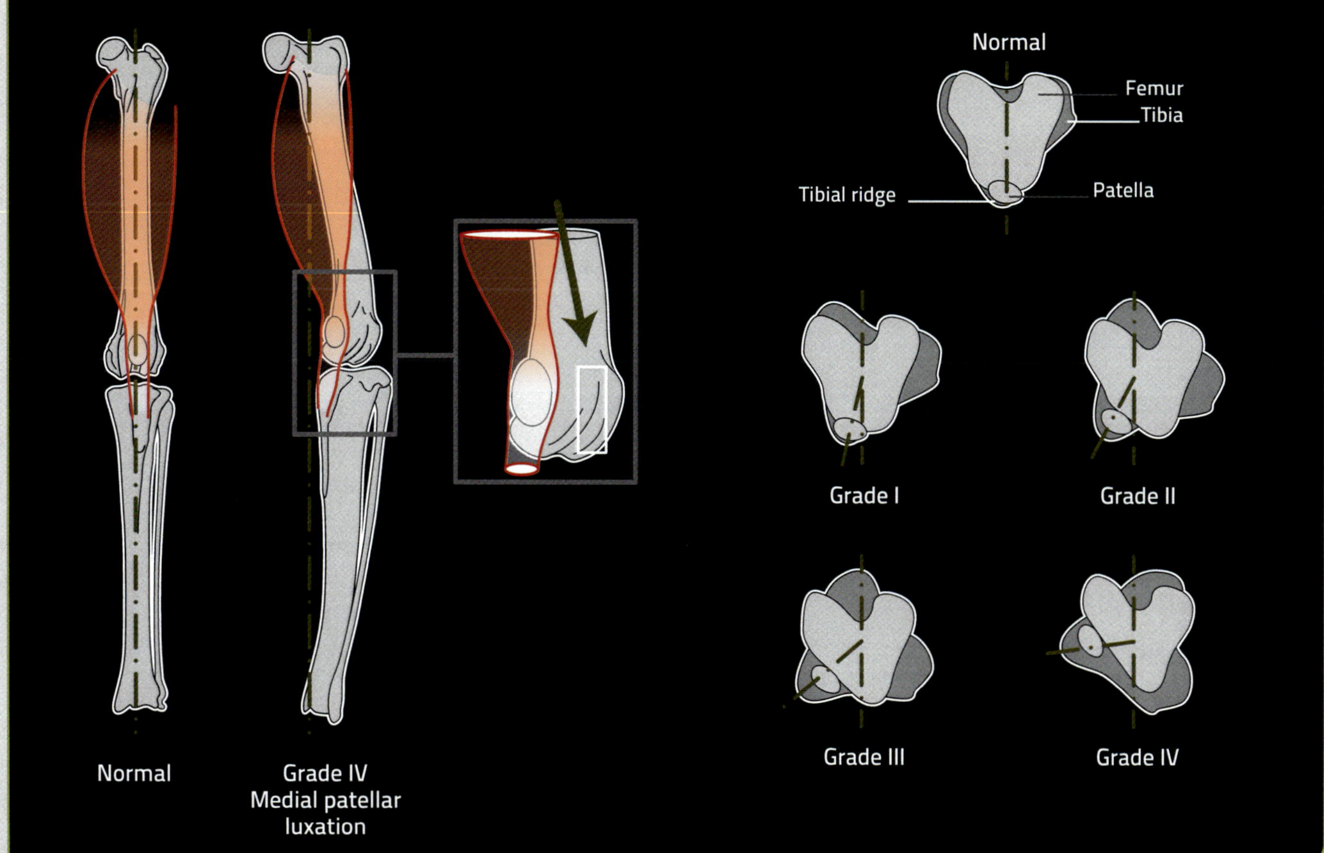

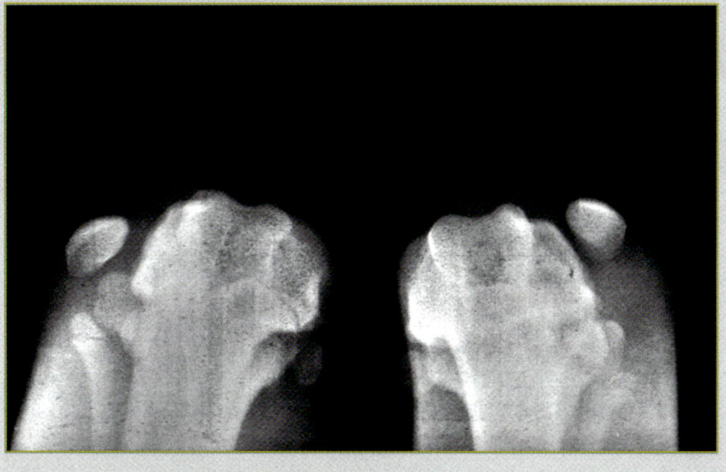

Figure 8. X-ray of maximum grade patellar luxation in a dog.

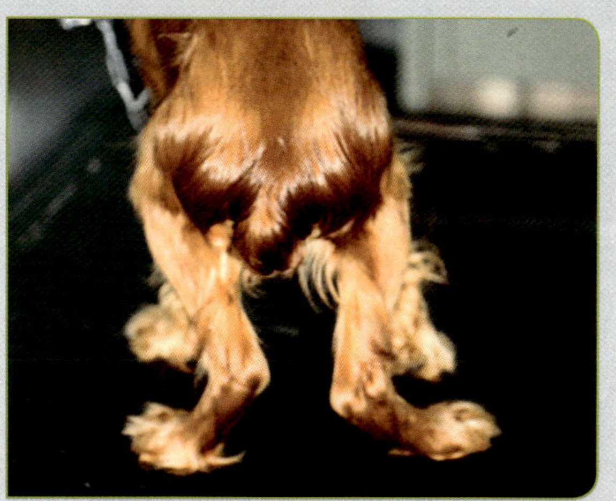

Figure 9. Cocker Spaniel with a lateral patellar luxation. The condition is bilateral, seen in the typical posture with semi-flexed limbs. The X-ray of this case is shown in Figure 8.

03 Osteochondrosis dissecans (OCD)

This condition is commonly found in giant breeds, and is particularly common in the German Shepherd. The first symptoms appear at 5-7 months. The stifle joint becomes inflamed, with pain on extension and muscular atrophy. Craniocaudal, caudocranial and mediolateral X-ray images are required for a clear diagnosis. The changes present are evident, and are always observed on the lateral condyle (Figs. 10-15).

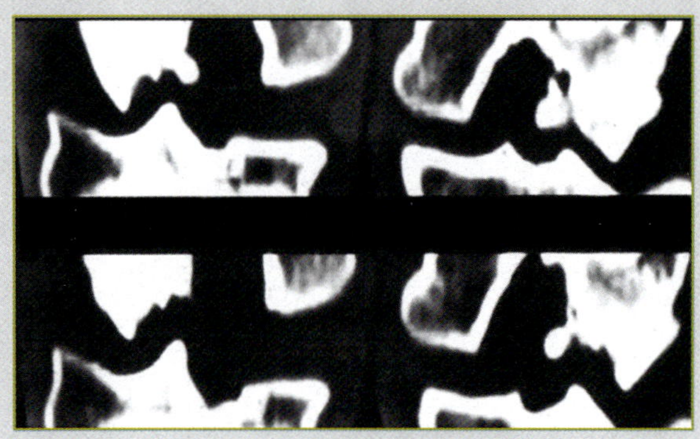

Figure 10. Different CAT sections showing the injuries.

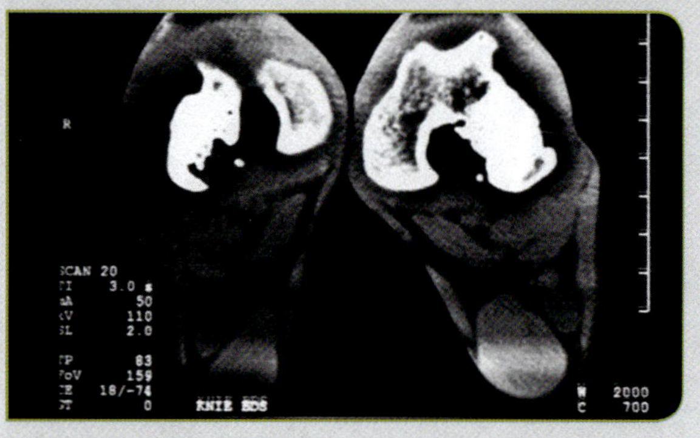

Figure 11. MRI of osteochondrosis dissecans, clearly showing an area of greater radio density on the lateral condyle.

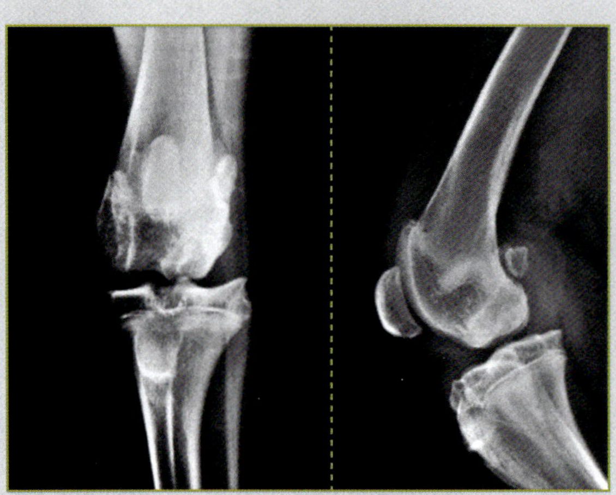

Figure 12. X-ray images showing alteration to the lateral condyle.

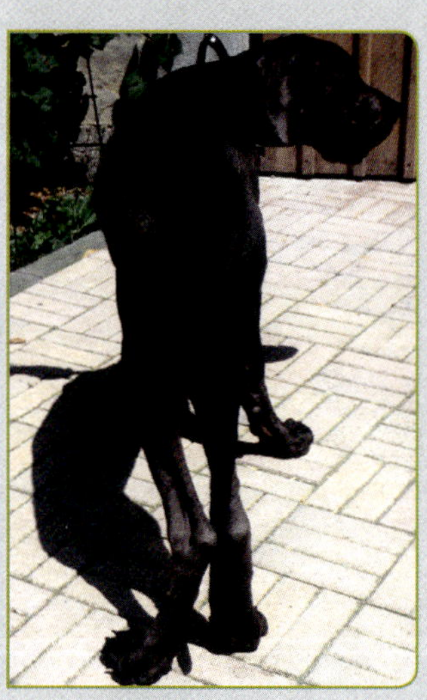

Figure 13. Typical posture adopted by animals suffering from OCD, bilateral in this case. This is a 9 month old Great Dane, clearly showing limb deformity, abduction of the stifle joints and closely positioned tarsals.

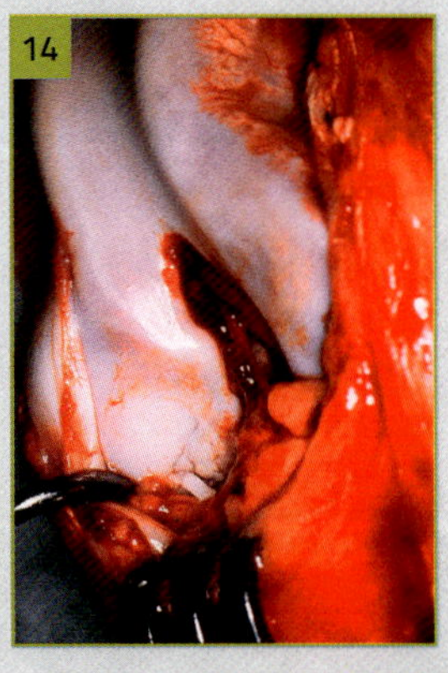

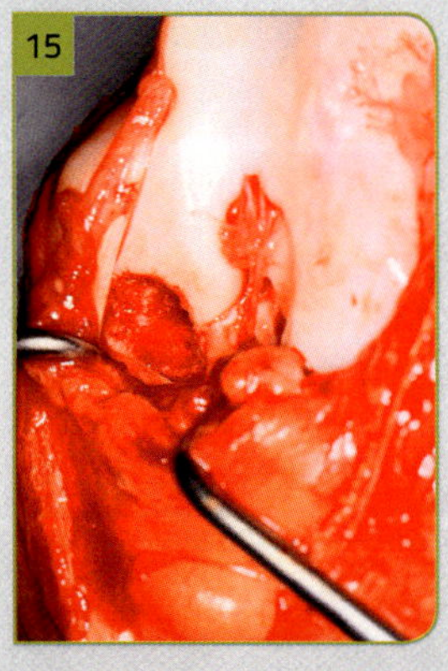

Figure 14. Image prior to curettage using the Pridie drilling technique. The damage is always on the lateral condyle.

Figure 15. Image of joint after surgery using the Pridie method, performed via a small hole drilled into the bed of the damaged cartilage, to allow the blood vessels of the subchondral tissue to regenerate the cartilage with fibrous tissue, rather than hyaline, which is the one present in this condition.

04 Arthritis/osteoarthritis

Isolated aseptic arthritis is unusual in small animals; polyarthritis is more common. Even more common is septic arthritis, caused by the administration of corticosteroid injections without taking the necessary antiseptic precautions. Treatment consists of joint lavage by arthrotomy, followed by immobilisation and antiinflammatory therapy (Figs. 16 and 17).

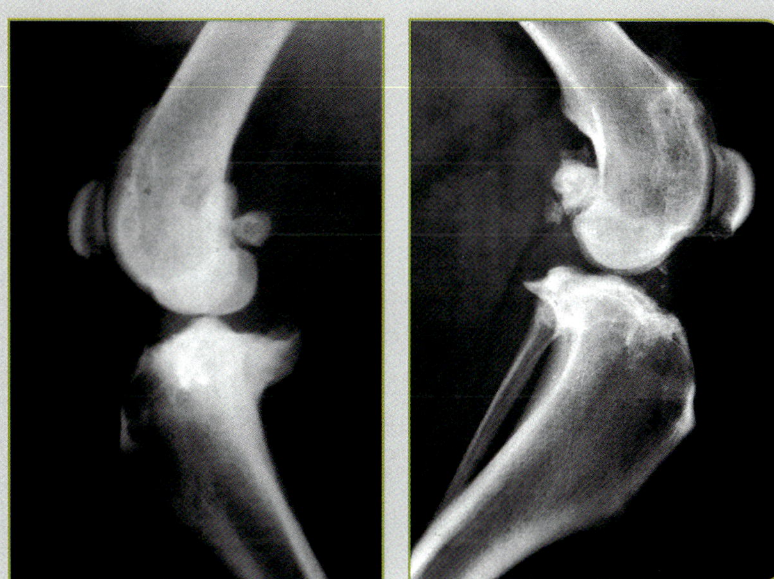

Figure 16. X-rays showing secondary osteoarthritis after rupture of the cranial cruciate ligament.

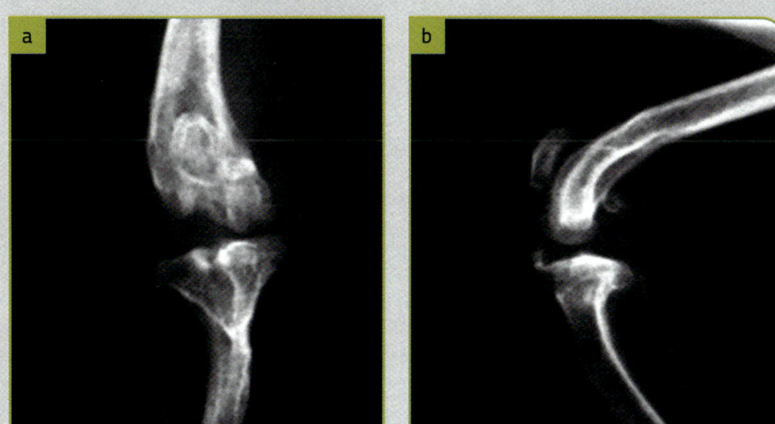

Figure 17. X-rays of severe osteoarthritis in a dog. Craniocaudal projection (a) and mediolateral projection (b).

Diagnostic imaging techniques

For the purposes of the first chapter only, below is a brief description of the most advanced diagnostic imaging techniques available, including illustrative examples of the stifle joint.

Computerised axial tomography

LATERAL VIEW

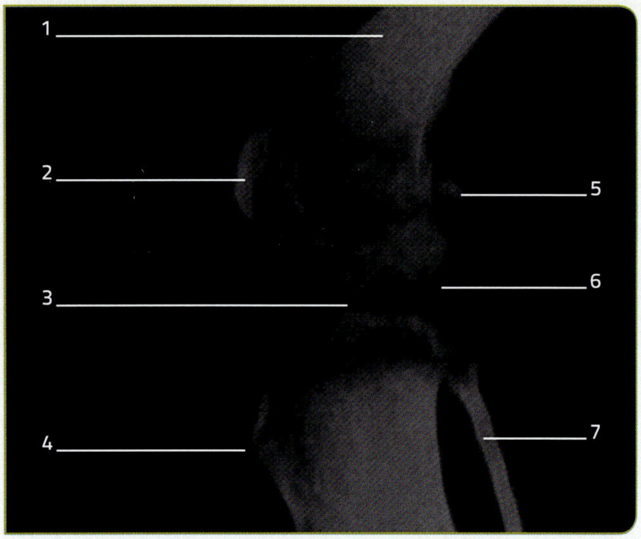

CRANIAL VIEW

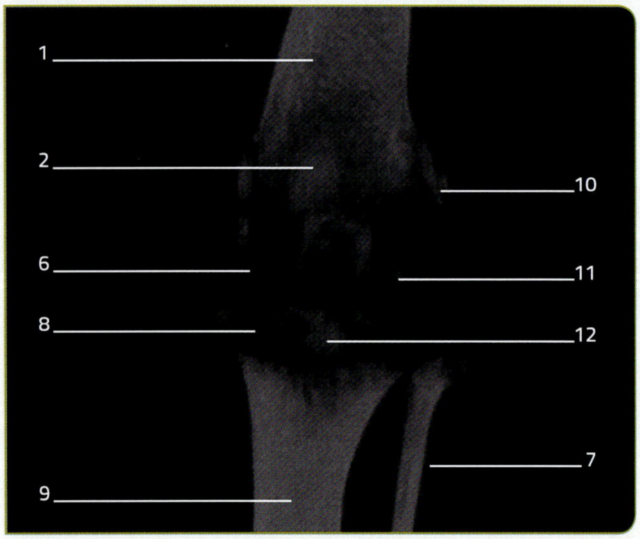

Computerised axial tomography (CAT) is a diagnostic imaging method that provides two- or three-dimensional images of the internal anatomical structures of the patient to facilitate a clear view of the body.

Using X-ray technology, different sections can be obtained from different angles, and then processed by a computer to generate images. With this technology, clinical studies can also be performed on the animal in a relatively short period of time, and in most cases under sedation only.

CAT scanning is increasingly common in veterinary medicine as it is of particular use in the study of pulmonary pathologies, the mediastinum, abdominal pathologies, vascular structures, oncology, neurology and the structures of the head. Furthermore, and increasingly so given the availability of 3D images, it is a useful tool in orthopaedics, as it provides high definition images for the examination of joints, fractures, etc.

1	Femur
2	Patella
3	Femorotibial joint
4	Tibial tuberosity
5	Gastrocnemius sesamoid bones
6	Medial femoral condyle
7	Fibula
8	Medial tibial condyle
9	Tibia
10	Lateral gastrocnemius sesamoid bone
11	Lateral femoral condyle
12	Popliteal notch

+ Watch this video on the electronic version
Computerised axial tomography

Fluoroscopy (angiography)

LATEROMEDIAL VIEW

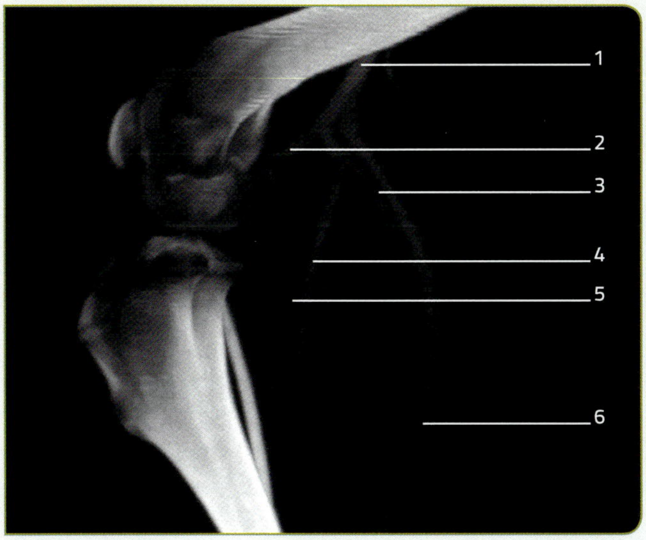

CRANIAL VIEW

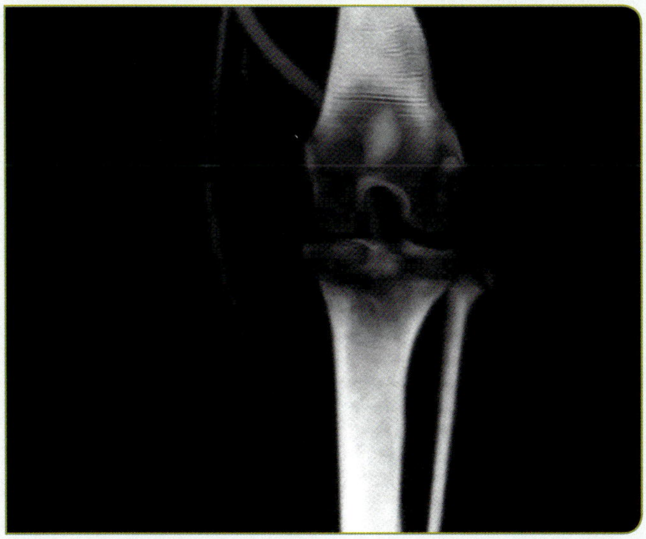

The use of fluoroscopy is becoming increasingly common in veterinary science; we can expect this X-ray imaging technique to eventually replace the traditional X-ray as a tool for diagnosis. However, ionising radiation must only be used where strictly necessary, and all required measures must be observed to ensure the safety of both the patient and veterinary surgeon.

The images obtained, depending on the technological capability of the equipment used, can be converted into videos or even three-dimensional images.

In addition to its use in orthopaedics, fluoroscopy is mainly used in the study of the digestive tract, urology and angiography.

1	Femoral artery
2	Popliteal artery
3	Distal caudal femoral artery
4	Medial saphenous vein
5	Saphenous artery
6	Lateral saphenous vein

Watch this video on the electronic version

Fluoroscopy - angiography

Three-dimensional computerised axial tomography

CRANIAL VIEW

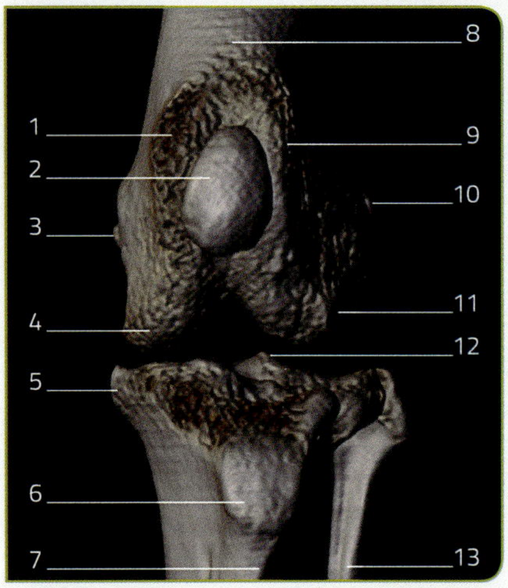

LATERO-LATERAL VIEW

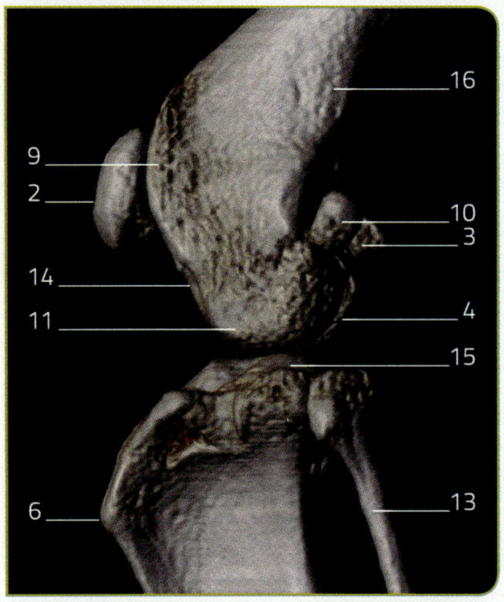

CAUDAL VIEW

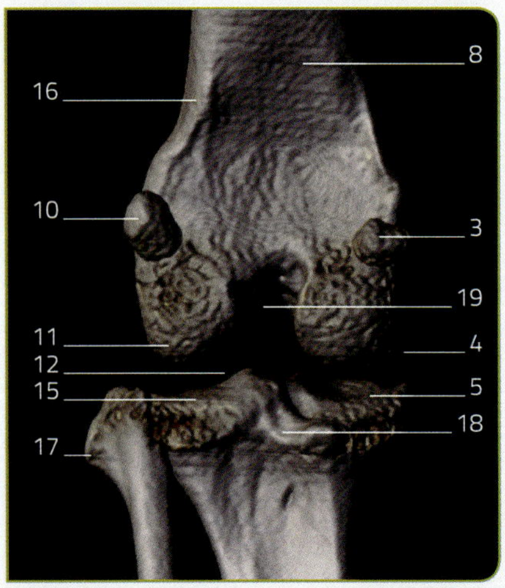

1	Medial ridge of the trochlea
2	Patella
3	Medial gastrocnemius sesamoid bone
4	Medial femoral condyle
5	Medial tibial condyle
6	Tibial tuberosity
7	Cranial border of the tibia
8	Femur
9	Lateral ridge of the trochlea
10	Lateral gastrocnemius sesamoid bone
11	Lateral femoral condyle
12	Lateral intercondylar eminence
13	Fibula
14	Extensor fossa
15	Lateral tibial condyle
16	Lateral supracondylar tuberosity
17	Head of the fibula
18	Popliteal notch
19	Intercondylar fossa of femur

Watch this video on the electronic version

Three-dimensional CAT

Three-dimensional computerised axial tomography + angiography

MEDIAL VIEW

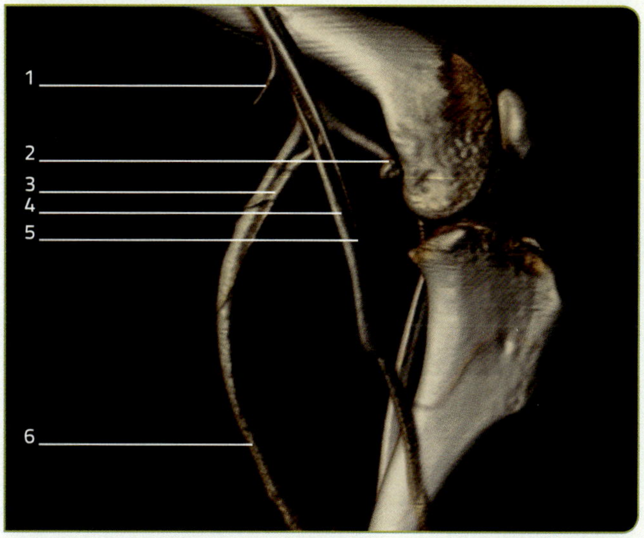

1	Middle caudal femoral artery
2	Popliteal artery
3	Distal caudal femoral artery
4	Medial saphenous vein
5	Saphenous artery
6	Lateral saphenous vein

CAUDAL VIEW

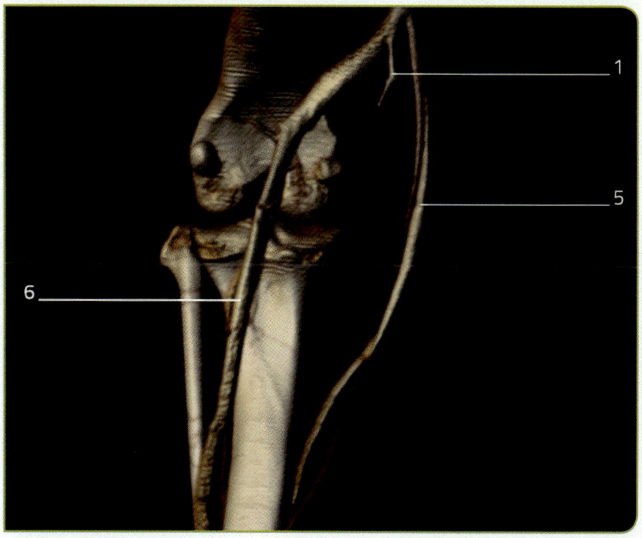

Watch this video on the electronic version

Three-dimensional CAT - angiography

Magnetic resonance

HORIZONTAL SECTION (PLANE) OF STIFLE JOINT **showing one of the cruciate ligaments**

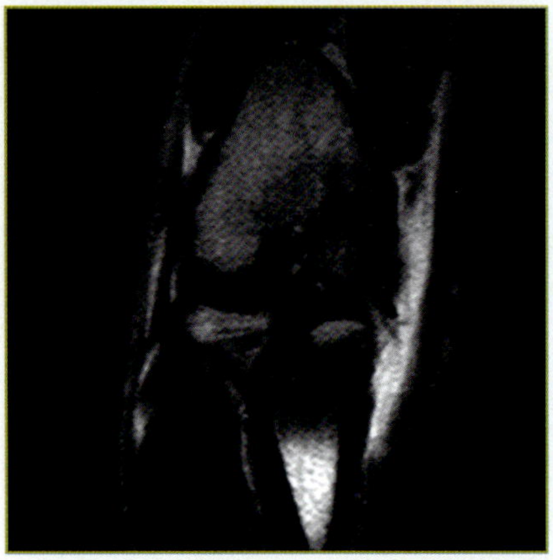

HORIZONTAL SECTION (PLANE) OF STIFLE JOINT **showing femoral and tibial articular surfaces**

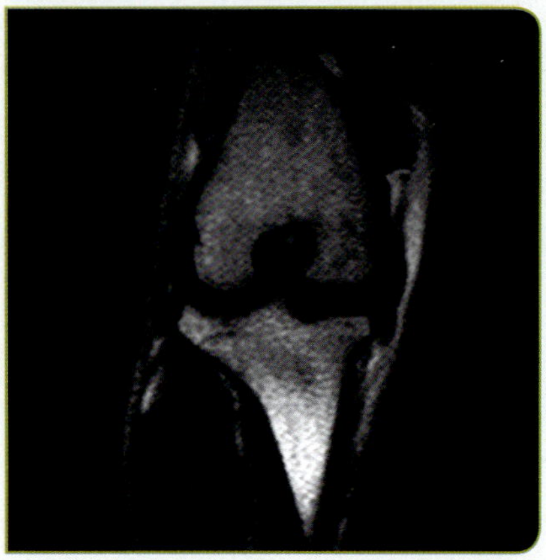

Nuclear magnetic resonance imaging (MRI) is a non-invasive diagnostic and exploratory technique that, unlike other methods such as CAT, does not use ionising radiation and processes data through a computer to obtain images from difference angles in real time.

Orthopaedics and neurology are the specialist areas that have benefited the most from this imaging technique, as it provides a detailed image of muscles and allows joints to be examined without surgery, and because it generates precise and risk-free images of the brain and spinal cord.

It can also be used when CAT scans are contraindicated and requires only mild anaesthesia or sedation, as the animal must be completely still for a period of time, depending on the examination performed.

The following are pairs of images comparing transparent plastinated sections of real structures compared with images obtained using CAT and MRI.

Transparent plastinated sections + CAT

SAGITTAL SECTION TAKEN AT THE INTERCONDYLAR FOSSA

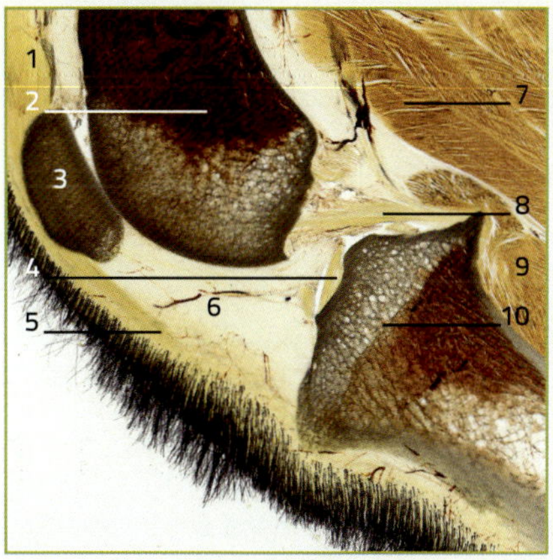

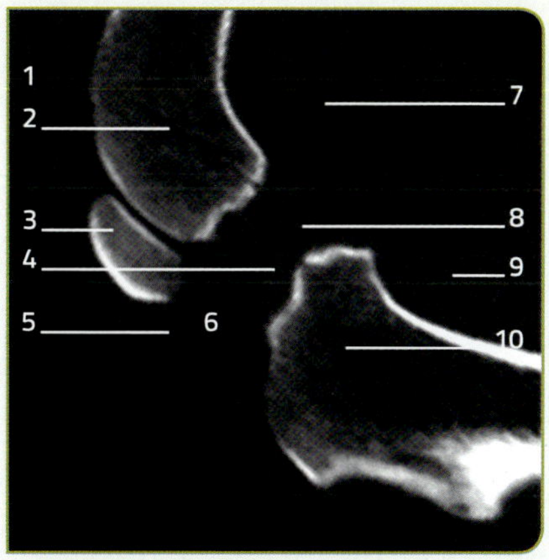

1	Quadriceps femoris tendon
2	Femur
3	Patella
4	Cranial cruciate lig.
5	Patellar lig.
6	Infrapatellar fat pad
7	Gastrocnemius muscle
8	Caudal cruciate lig.
9	Deep digital flexor muscle
10	Tibia

SAGITTAL SECTION TAKEN AT THE LATERAL FEMORAL CONDYLE

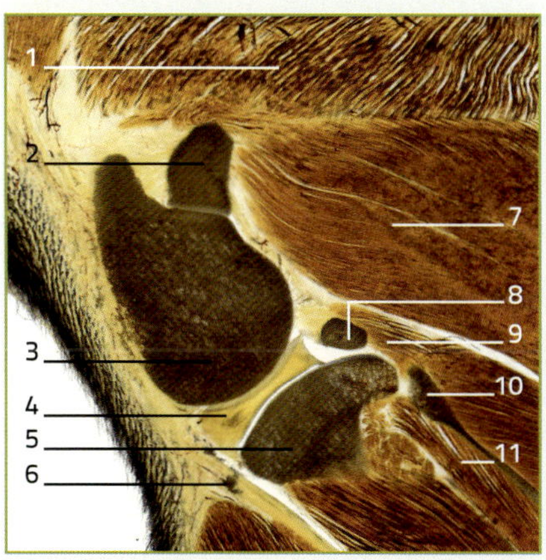

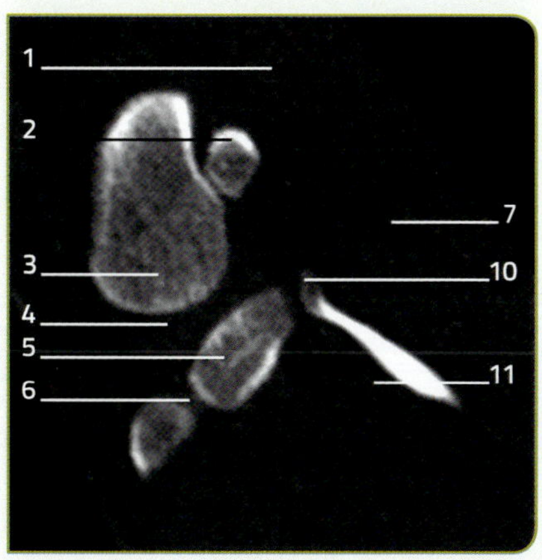

1	Biceps femoris muscle
2	Lateral gastrocnemius sesamoid bone
3	Lateral femoral condyle
4	Lateral meniscus
5	Lateral tibial condyle
6	Long digital extensor tendon
7	Gastrocnemius muscle, lateral head
8	Popliteus muscle sesamoid bone
9	Popliteus muscle
10	Head of the fibula
11	Lateral digital flexor muscle

Transparent plastinated sections + MRI

SAGITTAL SECTION TAKEN AT THE INTERCONDYLAR FOSSA

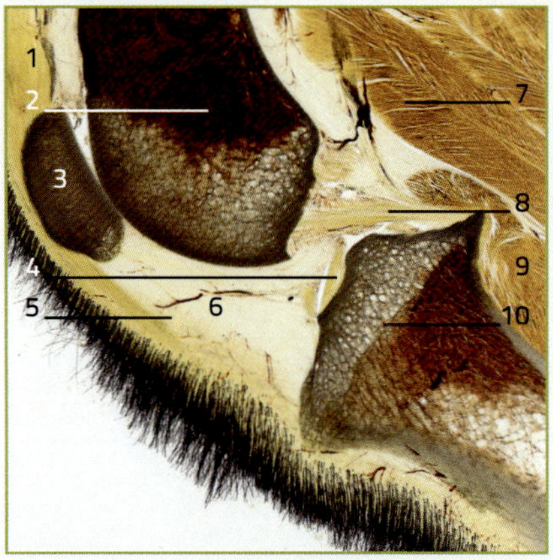

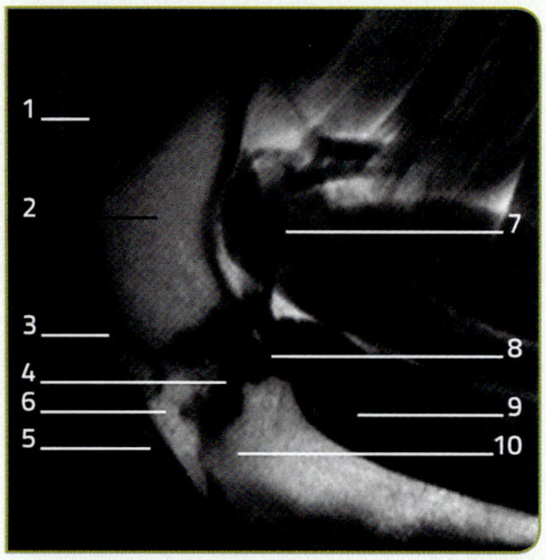

1	Quadriceps femoris tendon
2	Femur
3	Patella
4	Cranial cruciate lig.
5	Patellar lig.
6	Infrapatellar fat pad
7	Gastrocnemius muscle
8	Caudal cruciate lig.
9	Deep digital flexor muscle
10	Tibia

SAGITTAL SECTION TAKEN AT THE LATERAL FEMORAL CONDYLE

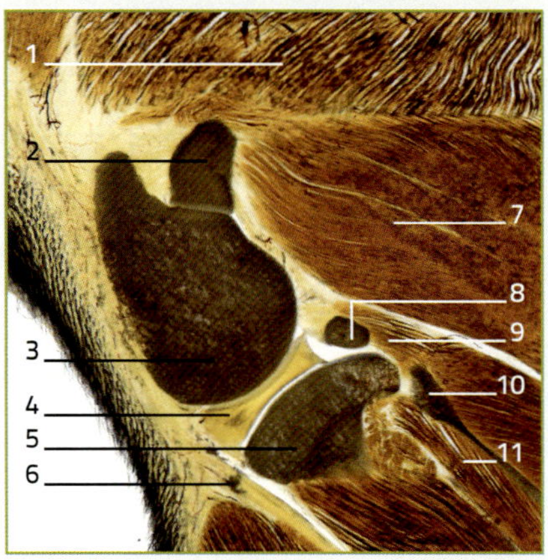

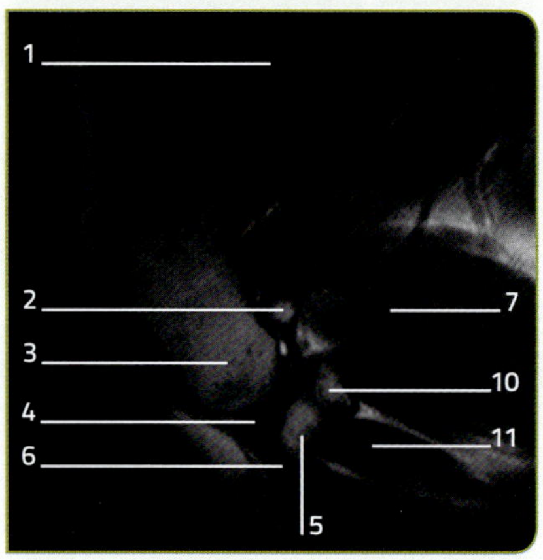

1	Biceps femoris muscle
2	Lateral gastrocnemius sesamoid bone
3	Lateral femoral condyle
4	Lateral meniscus
5	Lateral tibial condyle
6	Tendon of origin of the long digital extensor muscle
7	Gastrocnemius muscle, lateral head
8	Popliteus muscle sesamoid bone
9	Popliteus muscle
10	Head of the fibula
11	Lateral digital flexor muscle

SURGICAL APPROACHES

Approach to the distal portion of the femur and the stifle joint via lateral incision

1 With the animal in lateral recumbency, the incision is made in a curve from the distal third of the femur to the proximal end of the tibia, passing over the lateral femoral epicondyle.

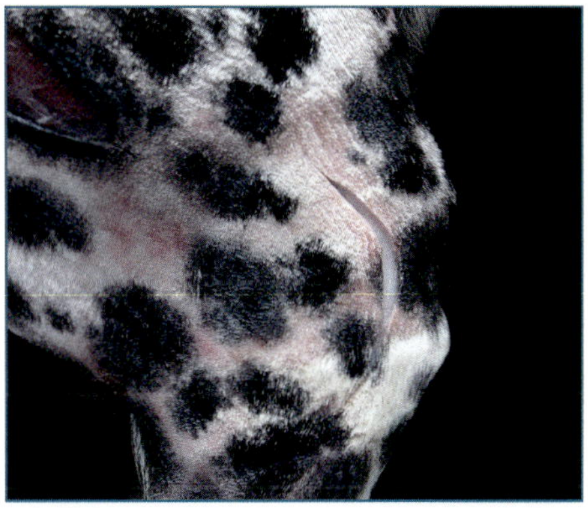

2 The stifle fascia is exposed and an incision is made in the aponeurosis of the biceps femoris muscle and the tendon of insertion of the quadriceps femoris, running parallel to the patella and patellar ligament.

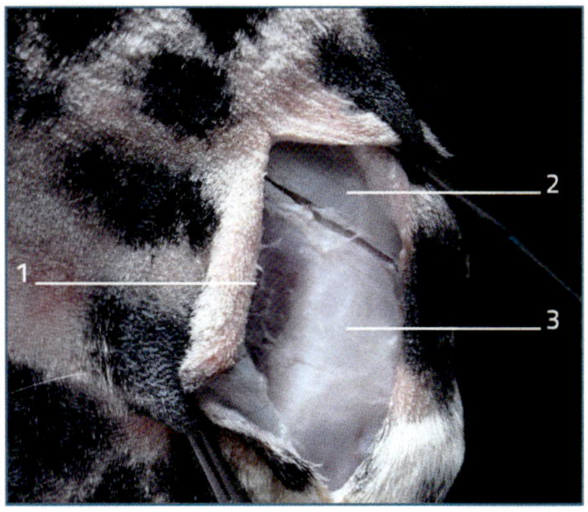

1 Biceps femoris muscle
2 Tendon of the quadriceps femoris muscle
3 Fascia lata

3 After sectioning the articular capsule, the quadriceps femoris tendon is displaced medially causing patellar luxation, thus exposing the interior of the joint.

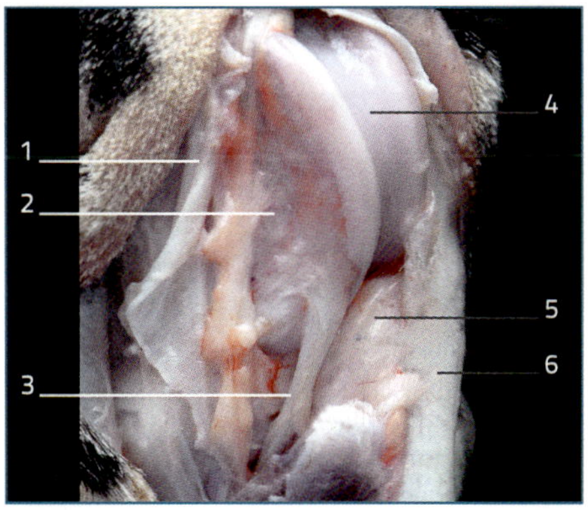

1 Articular capsule
2 Lateral femoral condyle
3 Long digital extensor tendon
4 Femoral trochlea
5 Infrapatellar fat pad
6 Patellar ligament

4 After forcing the joint into flexion the long digital extensor tendon and cranial and caudal cruciate ligaments can be observed, partially covered by the infrapatellar fat pad.

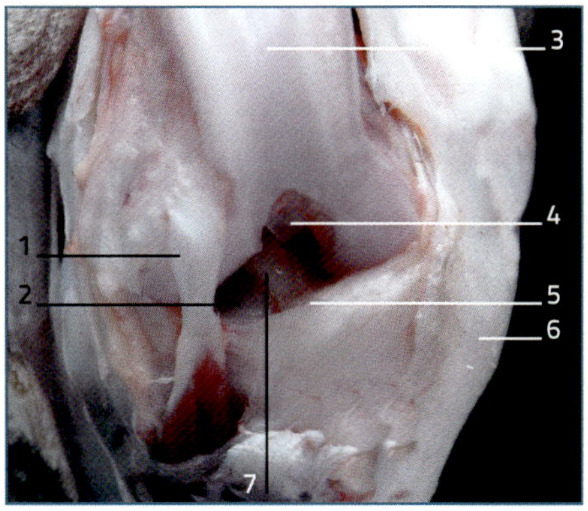

1 Long digital extensor tendon
2 Lateral meniscus
3 Femoral trochlea
4 Caudal cruciate ligament
5 Transverse ligament
6 Patellar ligament
7 Cranial cruciate ligament

Approach to the medial collateral ligament and the caudomedial region of the stifle joint

1 This approach requires lateral recumbency with abducted contralateral limb. The skin incision is made over the medial femoral epicondyle, extending proximally and distally in an arc.

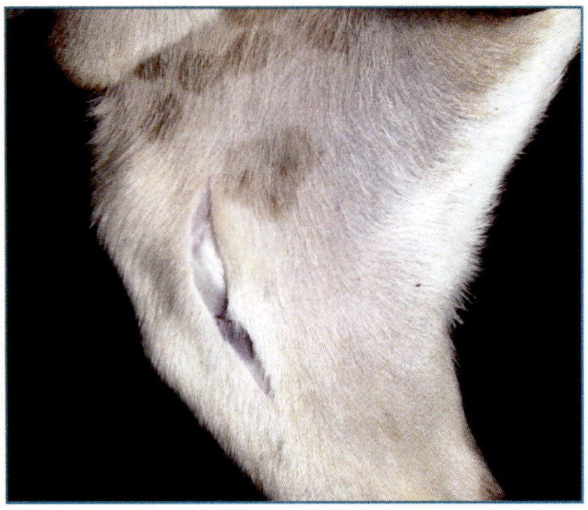

2 After partial resection of the stifle fascia, the insertion of the caudal portion of the sartorius muscle must be located and partially sectioned, taking care to avoid the descending artery and vein of the stifle joint.

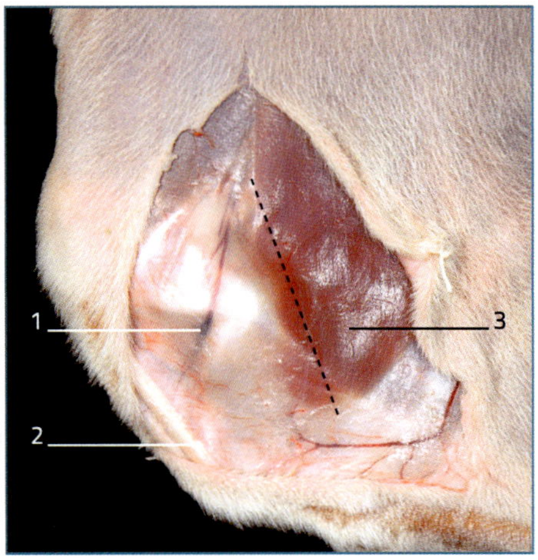

1 Descending artery and vein of the stifle joint
2 Patellar ligament
3 Sartorius muscle, caudal portion

3 After retracting the sartorius muscle caudally, the space between the insertions of the two portions of the semimembranosus muscle is located.

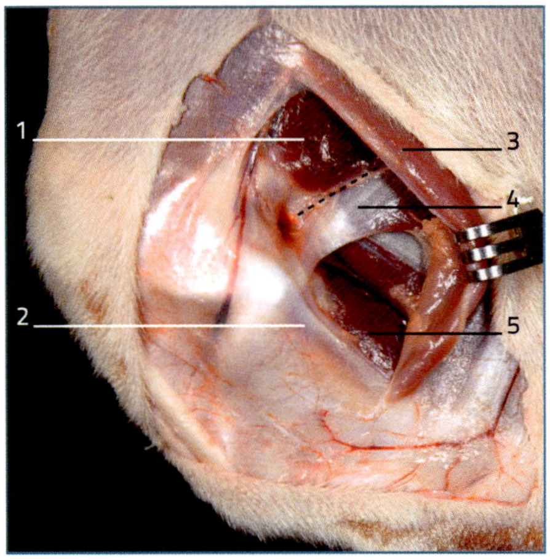

1 Semimembranosus muscle, cranial portion
2 Medial collateral ligament
3 Sartorius muscle, caudal portion
4 Semimembranosus muscle, caudal portion
5 Popliteal muscle

4 The separation of both portions of the semimembranosus muscle exposes the articular capsule, between the medial collateral ligament and the medial portion of the gastrocnemius muscle. After sectioning of the capsule the joint surface of the medial femoral condyle is located.

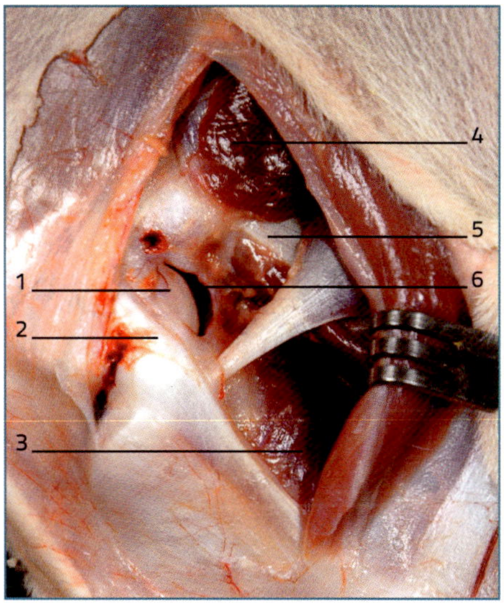

1 Medial femoral condyle
2 Medial collateral ligament
3 Popliteus muscle
4 Semimembranosus muscle, cranial portion
5 Gastrocnemius muscle, medial portion
6 Articular capsule

5 To observe the extension of the medial meniscus the tendon of insertion of the semimembranosus muscle (caudal portion) must be moved distally.

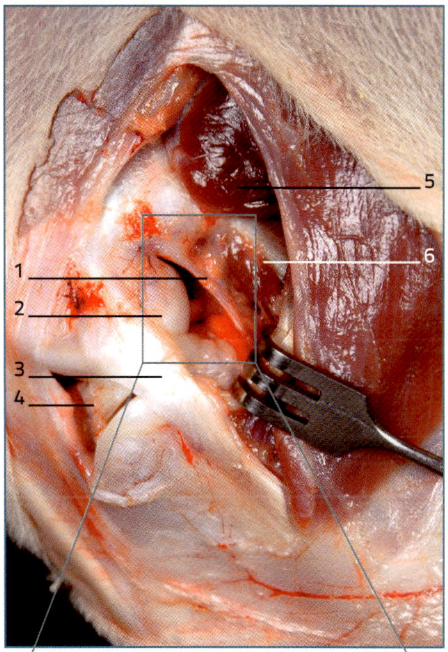

1 Articular capsule
2 Medial femoral condyle
3 Medial collateral ligament
4 Medial meniscus
5 Semimembranosus muscle, cranial portion
6 Gastrocnemius muscle, medial portion

6 The extension of the medial meniscus is located both cranially and caudally to the medial collateral ligament.

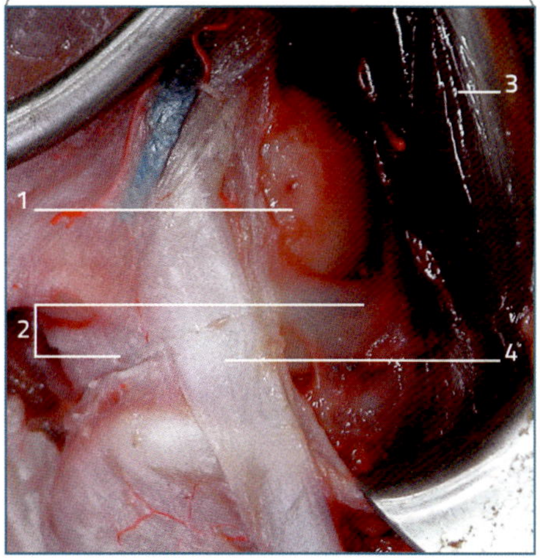

1 Medial femoral condyle
2 Medial meniscus
3 Gastrocnemius muscle, medial portion
4 Medial collateral ligament

Approach to the lateral collateral ligament and the caudolateral region of the stifle joint

1 The incision must run along the lateral epicondyle of the femur and extend in an arc proximally and distally.

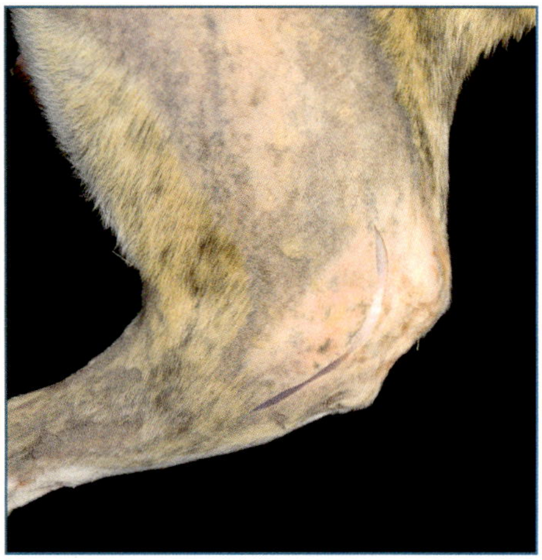

2 The vastus lateralis and biceps femoris muscles must be located and separated from each other along the course of the lateral collateral ligament.

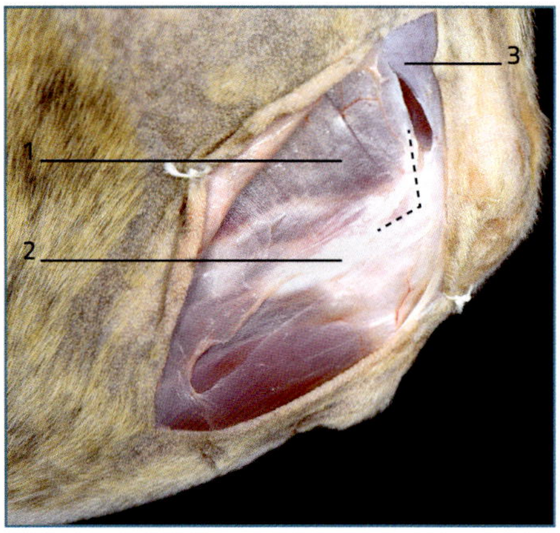

1 Biceps femoris muscle
2 Lateral collateral ligament
3 Vastus lateralis muscle

3 To locate the space between the gastrocnemius muscle (lateral head) and the lateral collateral ligament the biceps femoris muscle must be retracted caudally. It is important to take care not to damage the common fibular nerve.

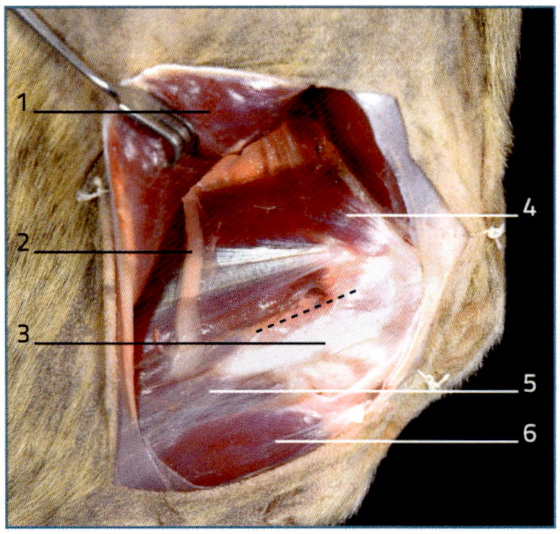

1 Biceps femoris muscle
2 Common fibular nerve
3 Lateral collateral ligament
4 Gastrocnemius muscle, lateral head
5 Long fibular muscle
6 Cranial tibial muscle

4 Here the articular capsule can be identified, together with the popliteal muscle tendon, partially covering the lateral meniscus.

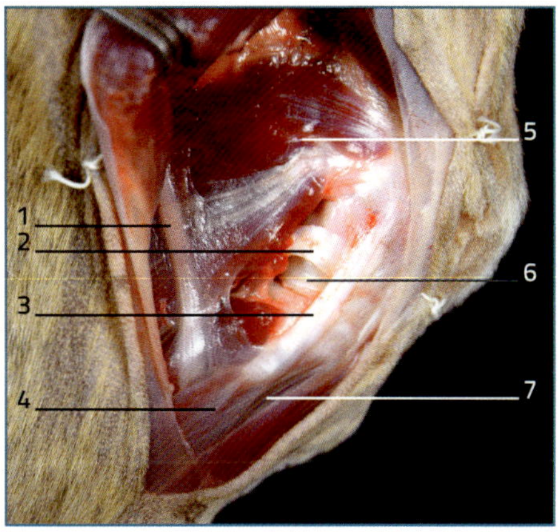

1 Common fibular nerve
2 Popliteal muscle tendon
3 Lateral collateral ligament
4 Long fibular muscle
5 Gastrocnemius muscle, lateral head
6 Lateral meniscus
7 Cranial tibial muscle

5 For a clearer view of the lateral meniscus, the popliteal muscle tendon must be displaced distally.

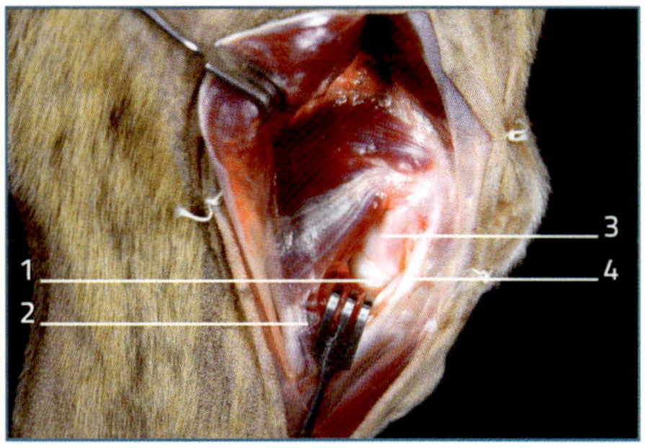

1 Lateral meniscus
2 Popliteus muscle
3 Lateral femoral condyle
4 Lateral collateral ligament

6 The position of the meniscus is limited laterally by the lateral collateral ligament.

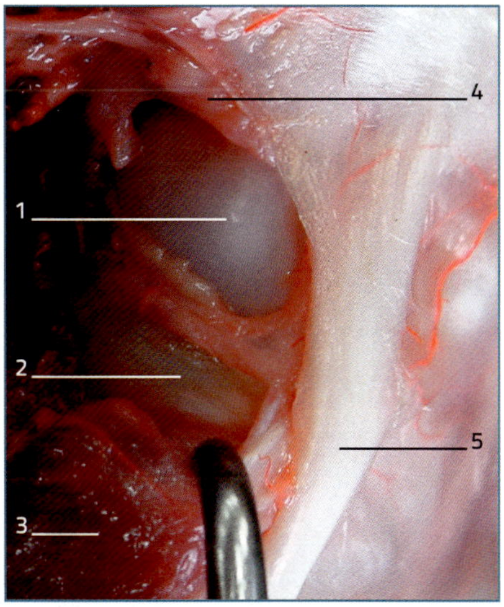

1 Lateral femoral condyle
2 Lateral meniscus
3 Popliteus muscle
4 Articular capsule
5 Lateral collateral ligament

Approach to the proximal portion of the tibia via medial incision

1 With the animal in lateral recumbency and the contralateral limb in abduction, an incision is made from the distal end of the femur to the medial surface of the tibia, passing over the medial femoral epicondyle.

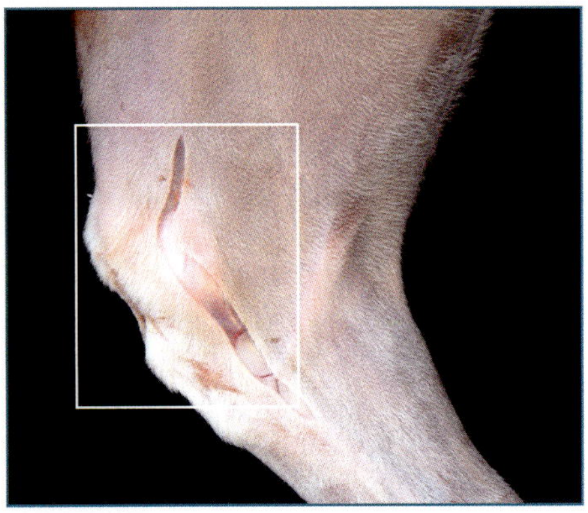

2 The aponeurosis of insertion of the caudal portion of the sartorius muscle must be sectioned caudally to the path of the medial collateral ligament, avoiding the descending blood vessels of the stifle joint.

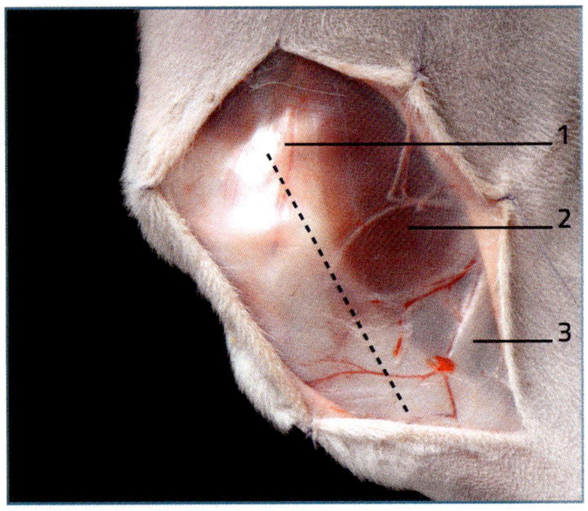

1 Descending artery and vein of the stifle joint
2 Sartorius muscle, caudal portion
3 Gracilis tendon

3 By displacing the sartorius muscle caudally, the tendons of insertion of the gracilis and semitendinosus muscles can be located in relation to the popliteus muscle.

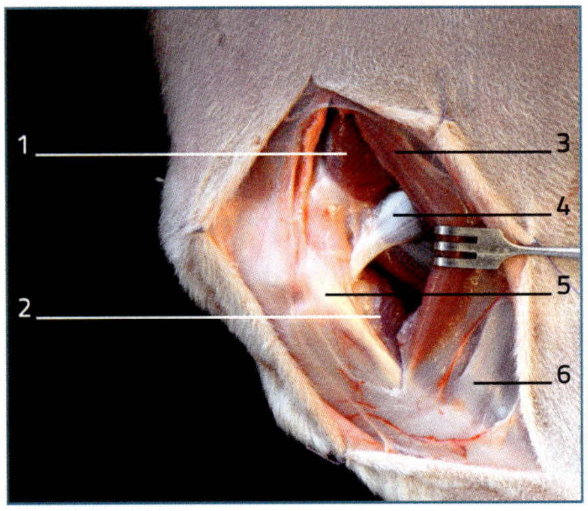

1 Semimembranosus muscle, cranial portion
2 Popliteus muscle
3 Sartorius muscle, caudal portion
4 Semimembranosus muscle, caudal portion
5 Medial collateral ligament
6 Gracilis tendon

4 The popliteus muscle is exposed by detaching the sartorius, gracilis and semitendinosus muscles. This exposes the entire insertion of the popliteus muscle at the medial edge of the tibia.

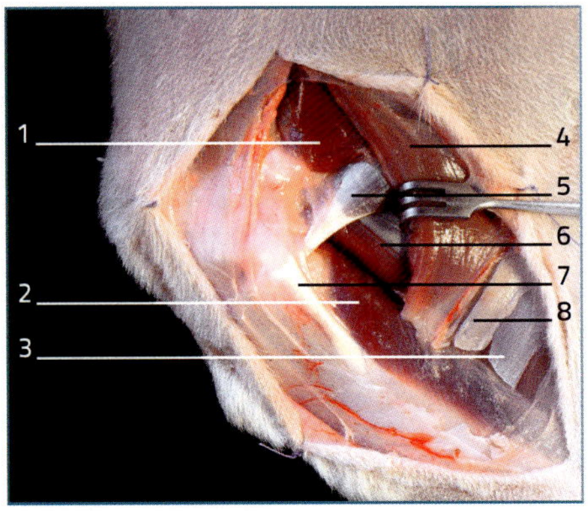

1 Semimembranosus muscle, cranial portion
2 Popliteus muscle
3 Semitendinosus tendon
4 Sartorius muscle, caudal portion
5 Semimembranosus muscle, caudal portion
6 Gastrocnemius muscle, lateral portion
7 Medial collateral ligament
8 Gracilis tendon

5 In order to expose the medial edge and the caudal surface of the proximal end of the tibia, the popliteus muscle must be detached and moved caudally. This procedure must be executed with care in order not to affect the popliteal artery and vein on their course through the popliteal notch of the tibia.

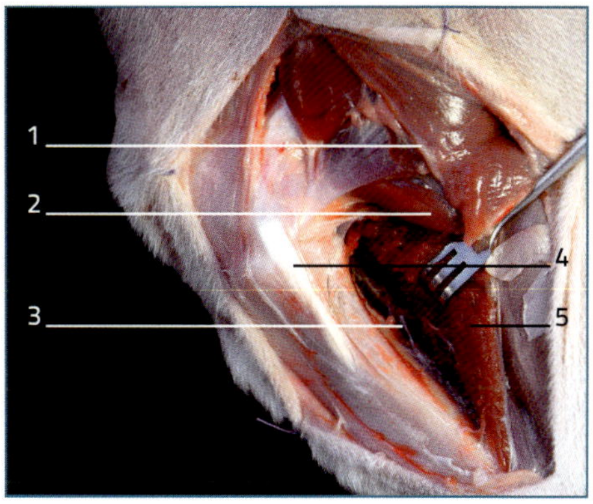

1 Sartorius muscle, caudal portion
2 Gastrocnemius muscle, lateral head
3 Popliteal artery and vein
4 Medial collateral ligament
5 Popliteus muscle

6 The tibial tuberosity is exposed by sectioning the cranial end of the fascia of the leg.

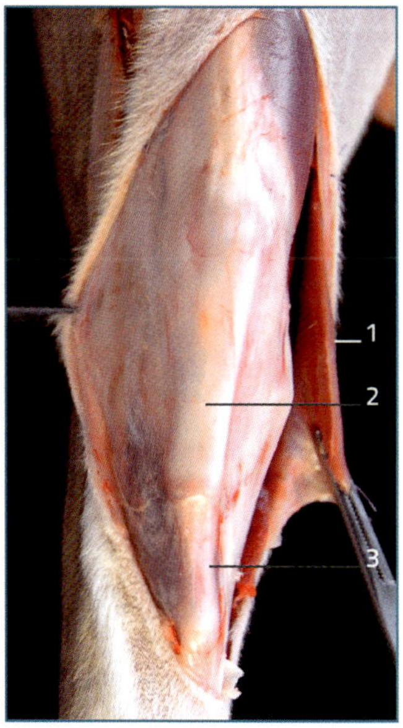

1 Sartorius muscle, caudal portion
2 Patellar ligament
3 Tibial tuberosity

7 To extend the approach towards the lateral area, the cranial tibial muscle can be detached from the tibial tuberosity.

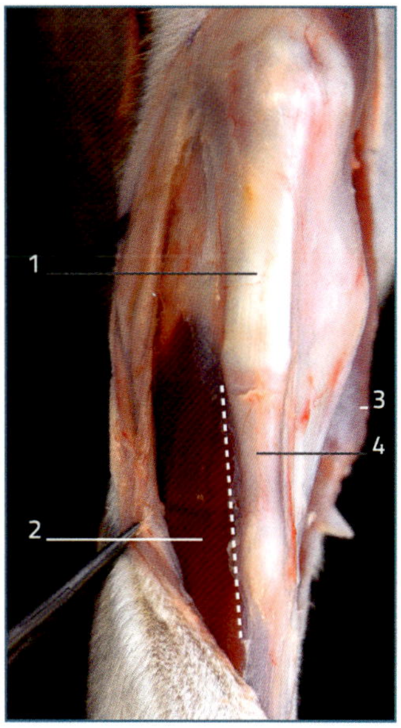

1 Patellar ligament
2 Cranial tibial muscle
3 Sartorius muscle, caudal portion
4 Tibial tuberosity

8 The procedure is completed by laterally retracting the remaining muscles, fully exposing the lateral surface of the tibia. It is important to respect the path of the long digital extensor tendon.

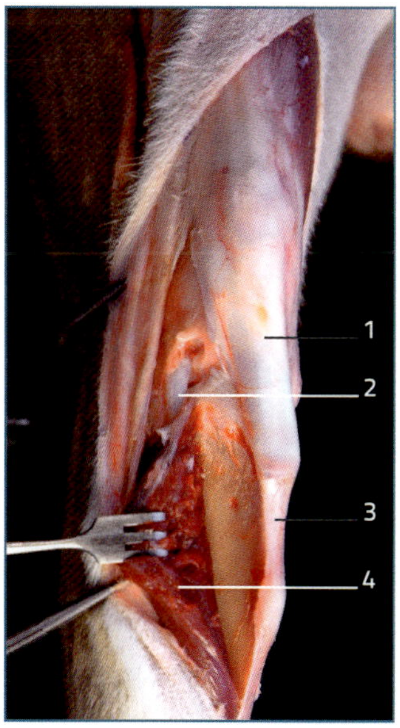

1 Patellar ligament
2 Long digital extensor tendon
3 Tibial tuberosity
4 Cranial tibial muscle

The images included for surgical approaches are adapted from: Latorre, R., Gil, F., Climent, S., López, O., Henry, R., Ayala, M., Ramírez, G., Martínez, F., Vázquez, J.M. *Color Atlas of Surgical Approaches to the Bones and Joints of the Dog and Cat*. Intermédica S.A., 2009; pp. 0-266. ISBN 978-950-555-353-2.

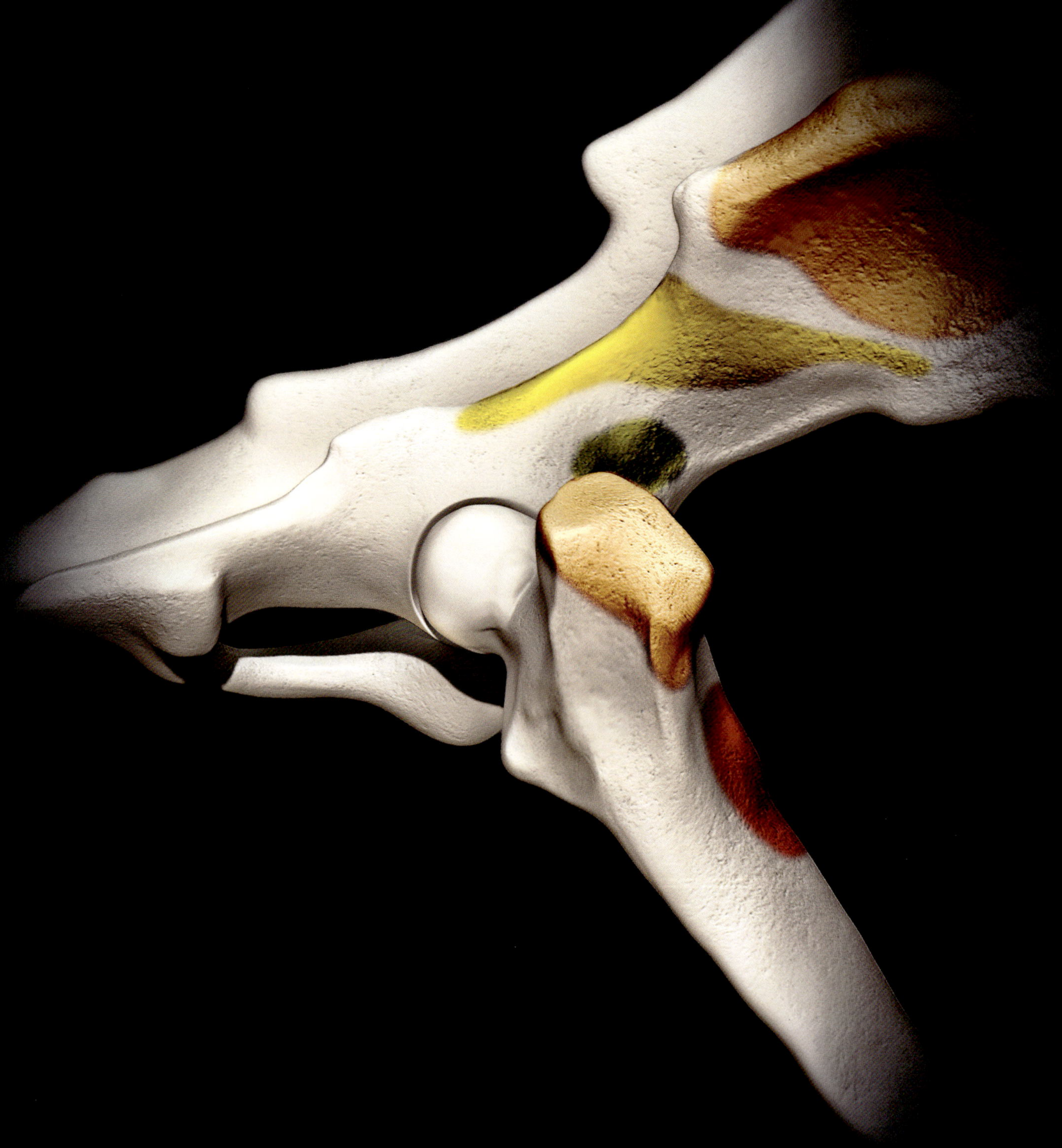

HIP JOINT

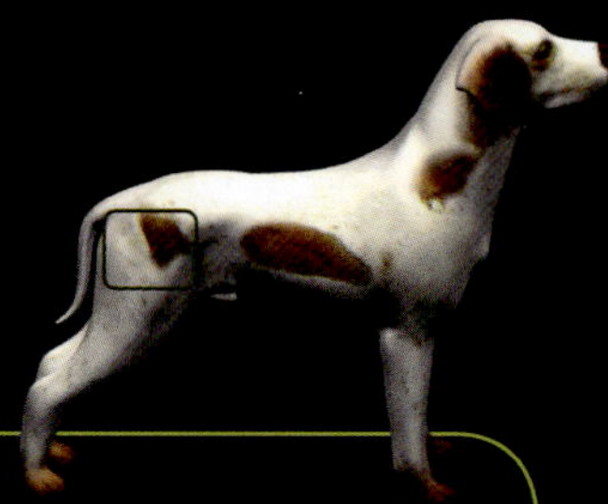

Hip joint

LATERODORSAL VIEW
IN ADDUCTION

Watch this video on the electronic version
Complete hip joint

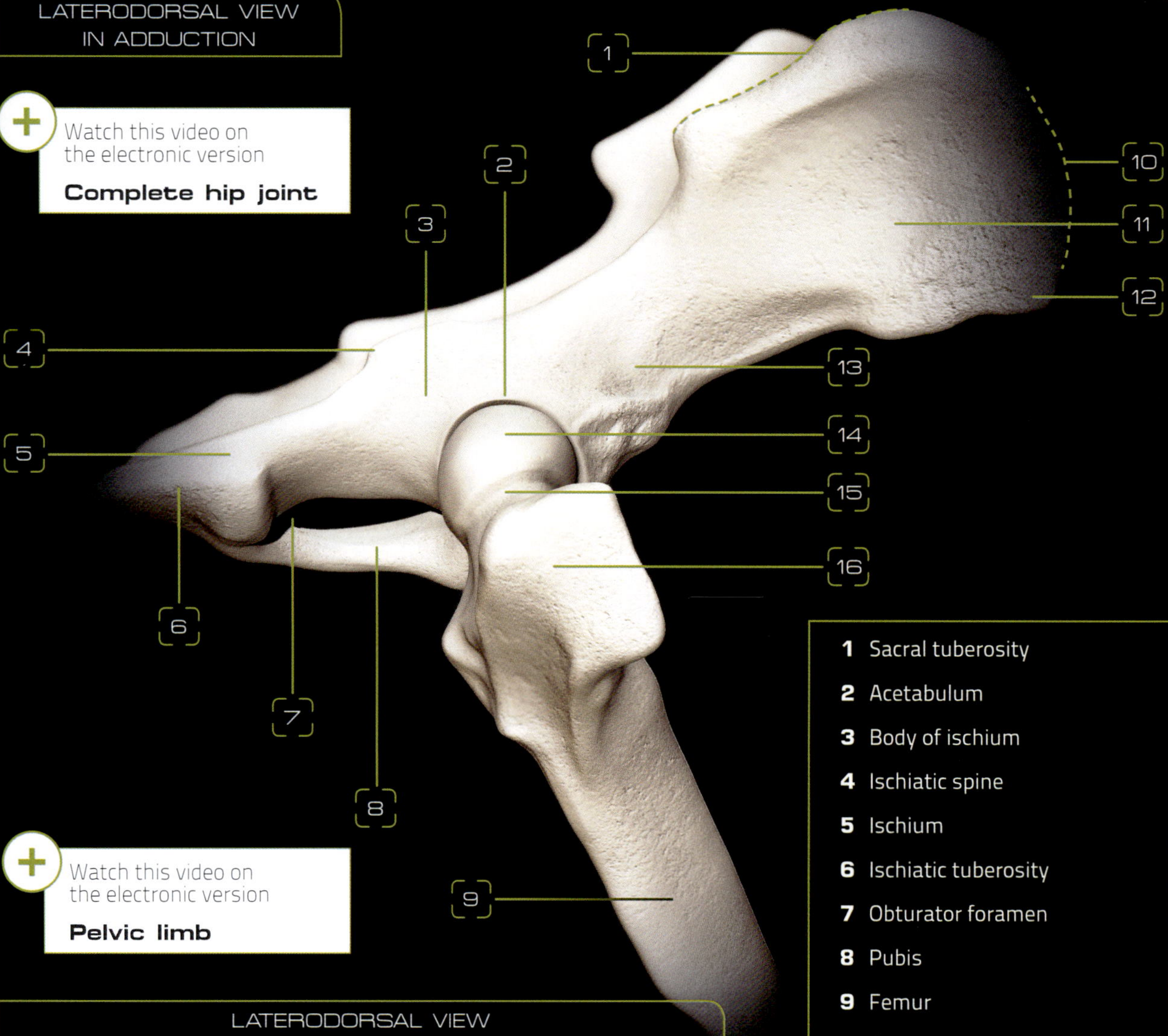

Watch this video on the electronic version
Pelvic limb

1 Sacral tuberosity
2 Acetabulum
3 Body of ischium
4 Ischiatic spine
5 Ischium
6 Ischiatic tuberosity
7 Obturator foramen
8 Pubis
9 Femur
10 Iliac crest
11 Wing of ilium
12 Coxal tuberosity
13 Body of ilium
14 Femoral head
15 Femoral neck
16 Greater trochanter
17 Acetabular fossa
18 Lunate surface of acetabulum
19 Transverse acetabular lig.
20 Lig. of head of femur
21 Acetabular fossa

LATERODORSAL VIEW
WITH DISTAL FEMORAL DISPLACEMENT

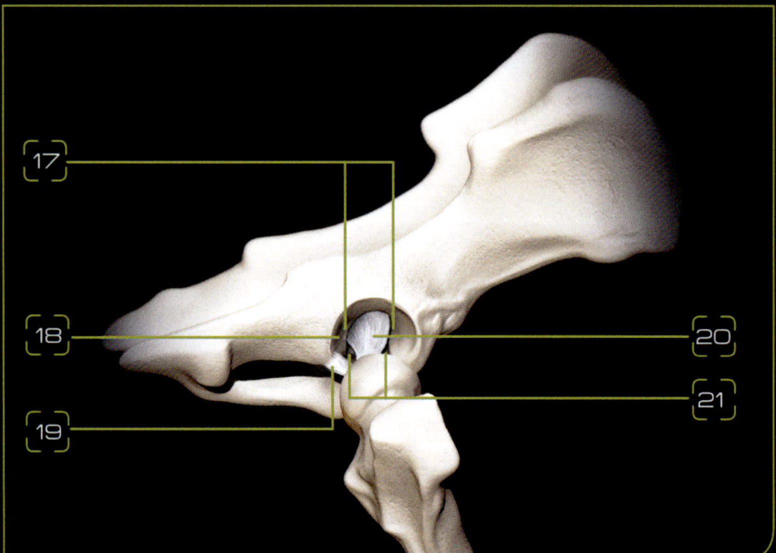

LATEROCRANIAL VIEW
WITH EXTERNAL FEMORAL ROTATION

1 Middle gluteal muscle
2 Superficial gluteal muscle
3 Deep gluteal muscle
4 Rectus femoris muscle

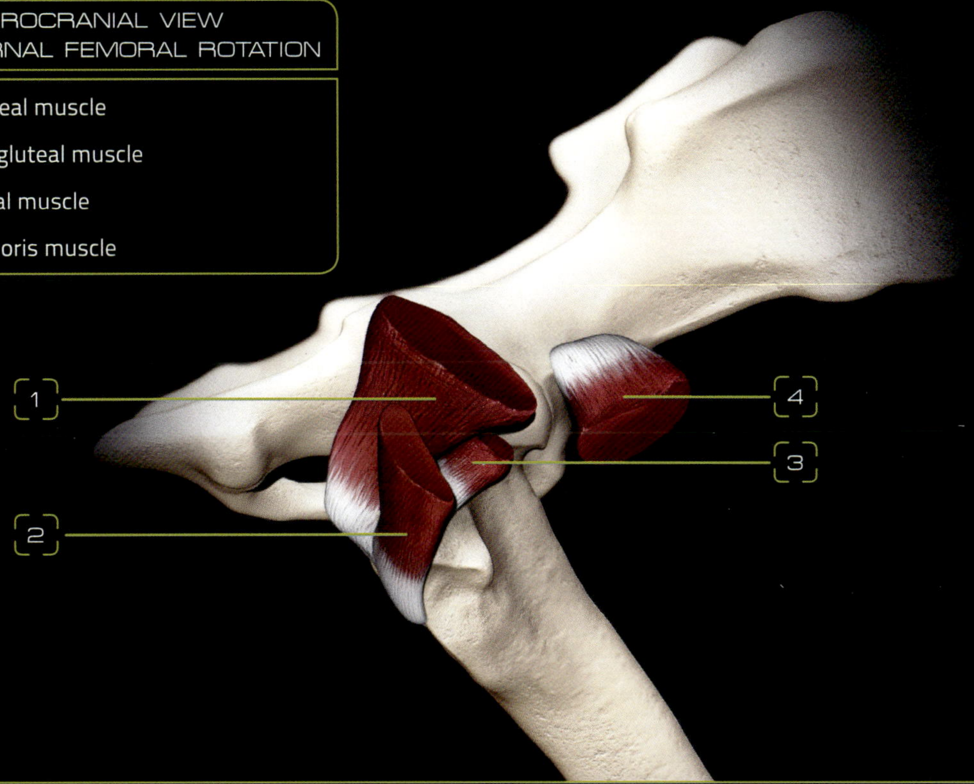

LATEROCAUDAL VIEW
WITH INTERNAL ROTATION OF FEMUR

1 Greater trochanter
2 Trochanteric fossa
3 Lesser trochanter

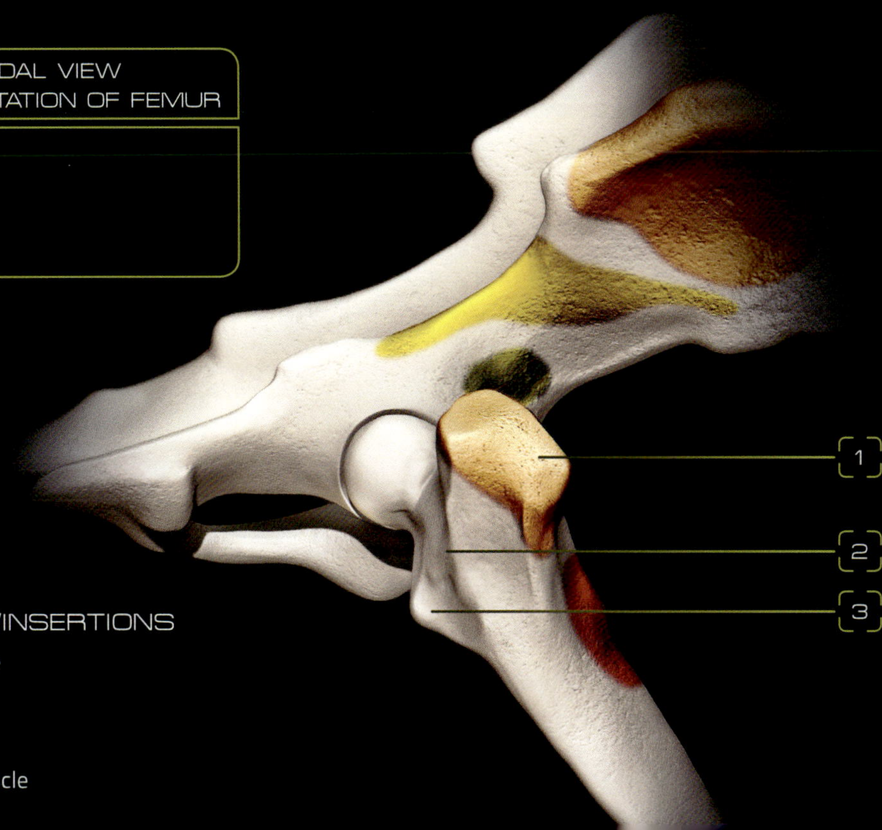

MUSCLE ORIGINS/INSERTIONS

- Rectus femoris muscle
- Deep gluteal muscle
- Middle gluteal muscle
- Superficial gluteal muscle

Orthopaedic conditions of the hip

In addition to fractures (not included in this work), the most common orthopaedic conditions of the hip joint are:

01 Hip dysplasia

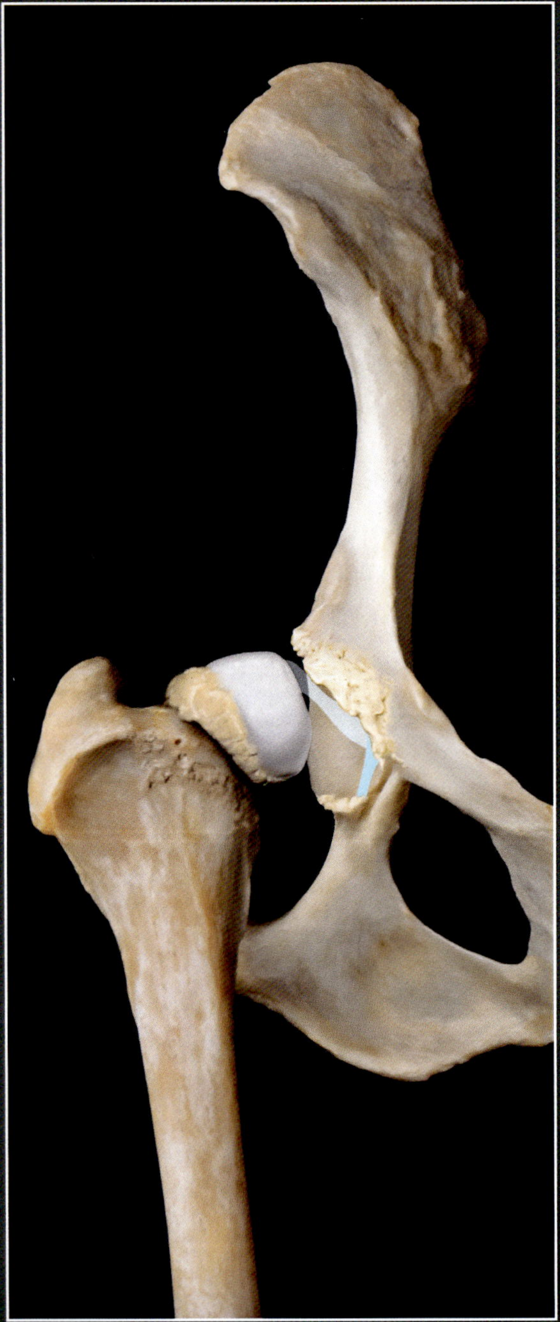

02 Avascular necrosis of the femoral head

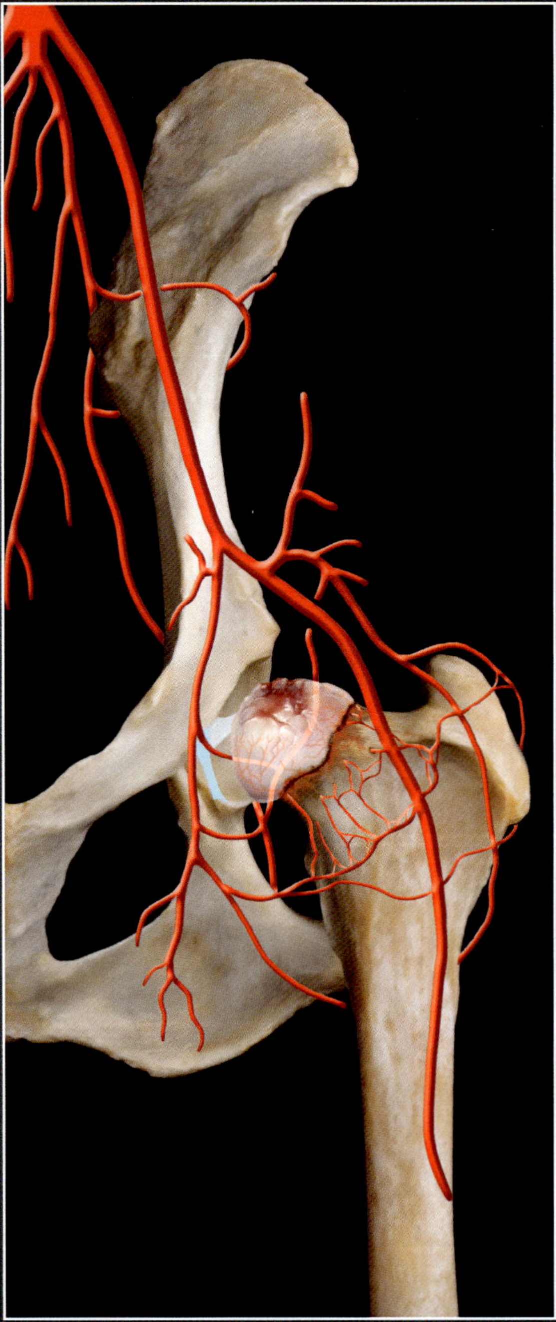

01

Hip dysplasia

It is important to stress the diagnosis of this pathology in young animals, as in adult dogs it is evident, so during clinical examination we must take particular care to identify the different aspects that accompany joint laxity in young dogs (Figs.1-4).

In order to make the correct decision regarding necessary treatment and prognosis, it is important to establish the severity of the different clinical signs of dysplasia in young animals. We must observe:

- The presence or absence of a well defined acetabular rim.
- Any deformity of the femoral head.
- Tension of the pectineus muscle.
- The angle of inclination and anteversion.

During the clinical examination of dogs with suspected hip dysplasia, no signs of alteration to the pelvic limb must be disregarded; and each one considered in minute detail. We must take note all possible discomfort, inability to climb, walk, or simply to remain standing for an extended period.

Clinical signs

The main symptoms we may find in a young dog are: difficulty remaining in a standing position (Fig. 5), walking or climbing stairs, and valgus deformity in the distal region of the limb. We must bear in mind that lameness may occur in one or both hind limbs and that exercise aggravates lameness or causes onset where it was not previously present. In general, dysplastic puppies always show greater intolerance to exercise than healthy puppies.

They present sudden onset weight-bearing lameness on a supported limb, without any previous trauma. The lameness may even disappear for variable periods of time - months or even years - but we must remember that the degenerative condition continues to progress, and if an early diagnosis is not established, these animals may cease to be eligible for surgical procedures such as TPO (Triple Pelvic Osteotomy) and may require other techniques such as prosthetics.

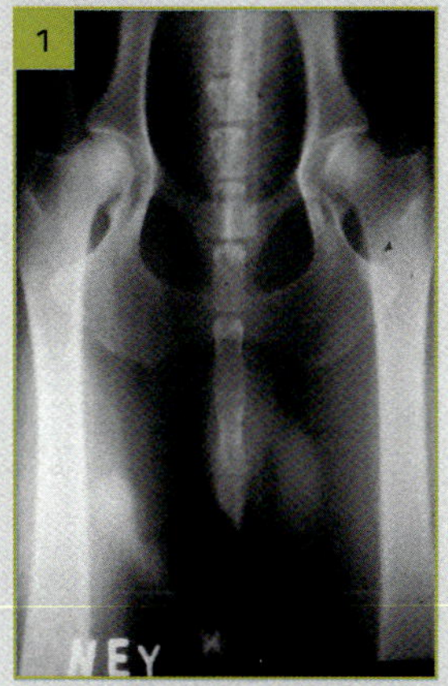

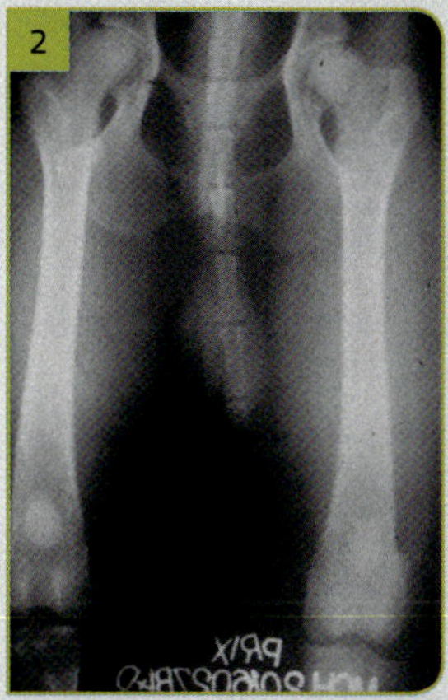

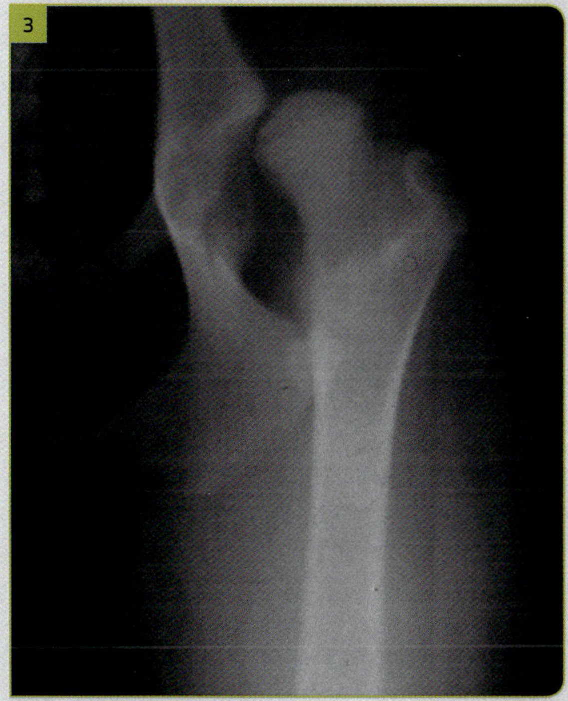

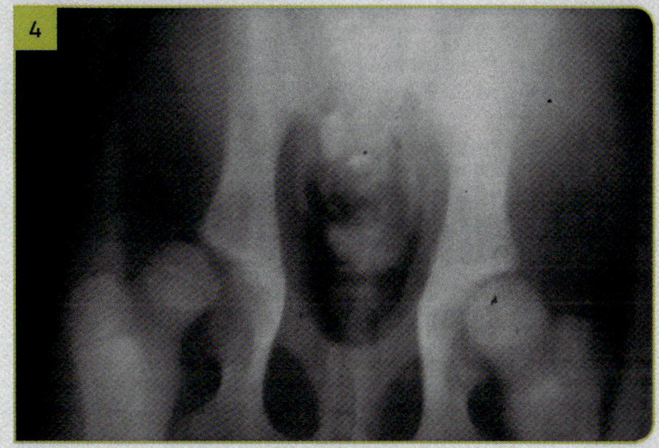

Figure 1. X-ray of a dog with hips in a normal position.
Figure 2. Well positioned hip joint.
Figure 3. Hip dysplasia.
Figure 4. Severe dysplasia in a puppy.

In young dogs, the joint presents synovitis with a distended joint capsule caused by synovial effusion, elongation and occasionally of the femoral head ligament, and micro-fractures and erosion along the cranial acetabular rim.

As the animal grows older, all this results in an increase in clinical symptoms and the onset of a degenerative joint condition that will continue to progress.

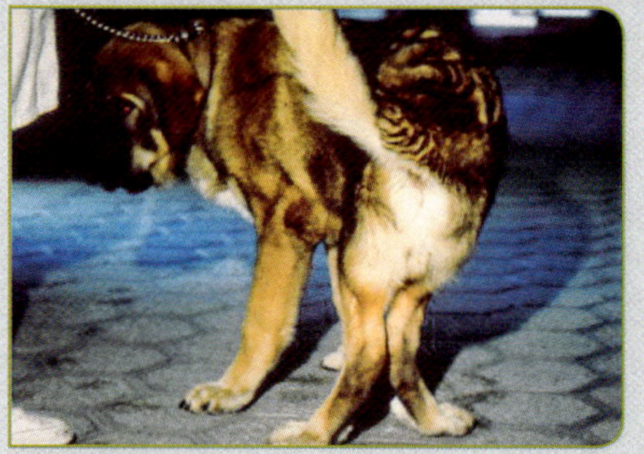

Figure 5. Clinical appearance of an animal with severe dysplasia.

Differential diagnosis

Hip dysplasia is a condition with no characteristic symptoms. Indeed, similar signs and symptoms of other conditions often lead to a misdiagnosis of dysplasia. A differential diagnosis must always be completed for comparison with other orthopaedic and neurological conditions (Table 1).

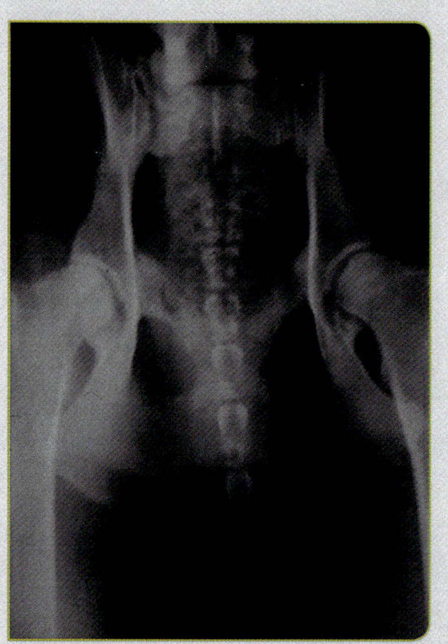

Figure 6. Cancerous lesion on the femoral head.

Table 1. Differential diagnosis of hip dysplasia.

Orthopaedic conditions

- Panosteitis.
- Osteochondrosis dissecans, both in the hip, stifle and tarsal joints.
- Patellar luxation.
- Hypertrophic osteodystrophy.
- Autoimmune diseases.
- Bone tumours (Fig. 6).
- Rupture of cranial cruciate ligament.

Neurological diseases

- Disc hernation.
- Cauda equina.
- Myelitis.
- Osteomalacia.
- Spinal tumours.

Physical examination

The animal must be first be examined and observed standing, walking and trotting.

With the dog in a standing position, the caudal third must be examined, observing the symmetry between the two hind limbs.

With the dog in lateral recumbency, we proceed to examine the limbs, searching for painful areas from the toes to the hip. We must also look for muscular atrophy, crepitation, clicking, loss of joint movement, the position of the greater trochanter and the presence of joint laxity (Fig. 7).

In dysplastic dogs eligible for surgery we can observe pain on extension and abduction of the affected limb. Orthoarthritic changes and fibrosis in the joint capsule and the surrounding muscles will result in a reduced ability for extension.

Joint laxity in young dogs (under 6 months) can be tested using the Ortolani or Barden tests, although at times the results are not clear.

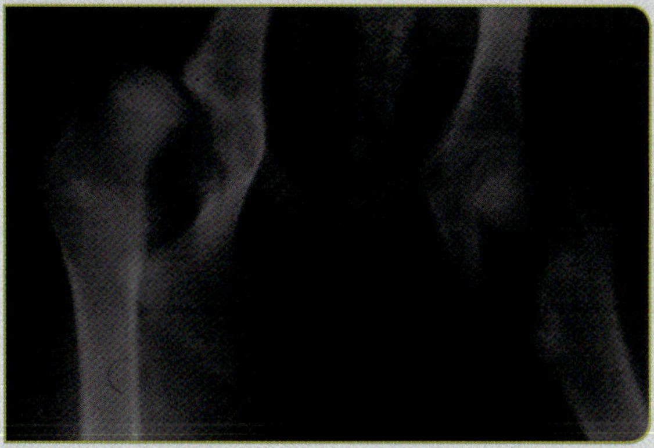

Figure 7. Severe dysplasia with subluxation.

For the Barden test, with the dog in lateral recumbency, stand behind the animal placing the thumb on the greater trochanter and the rest of the hand over the hip joint. With the other hand, push the quadriceps upwards. If the trochanter moves towards you, there is laxity in the joint. A deviation of half a centimetre is considered a positive result for this test.

It should be remembered that not all dysplastic dogs will obtain a positive result for these tests. An X-ray is always required in order to establish a firm diagnosis of this condition. For young dogs, a compression/distraction X-ray method can be used to obtain a mathematical calculation of joint laxity.

Ortolani test

This is performed with the animal under anaesthetic or deeply sedated, as it is very painful. It can be performed with the animal in lateral or dorsal recumbency:

- In **lateral recumbency**, with the femur horizontally, axial pressure is exerted at a 90° angle to the spine. If there is joint laxity the femoral head will luxate dorsally. Once in this position the limb is abducted, and if there is laxity of the femoral head it will return to the acetabulum, with a characteristic click.
- When performed in **dorsal recumbency** both femurs are positioned perpendicular to the table, and pressure is exerted through the stifle joints perpendicular to the table and the dog's spine. If there is joint laxity, dorsal subluxation of the femoral head will occur. Abduction will then return the femoral head to its correct position, with the characteristic click.

Two different types of angle are obtained in this test:

- **Angle of luxation**; the angle between the vertical and the point of adduction at which the femoral head subluxates.
- **Angle of reduction**; the angle between the vertical and the point of abduction where the femoral head returns to the acetabulum.

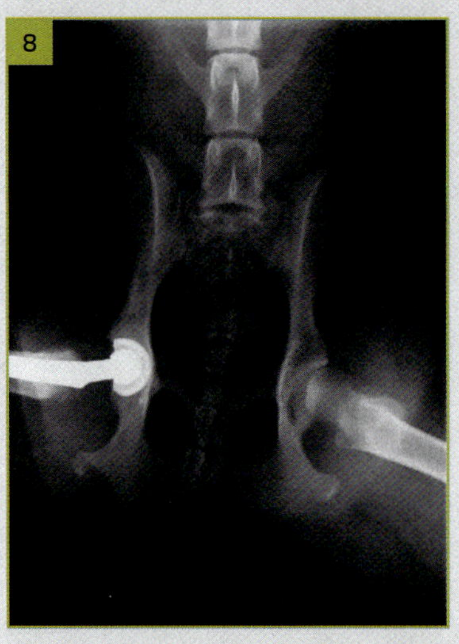

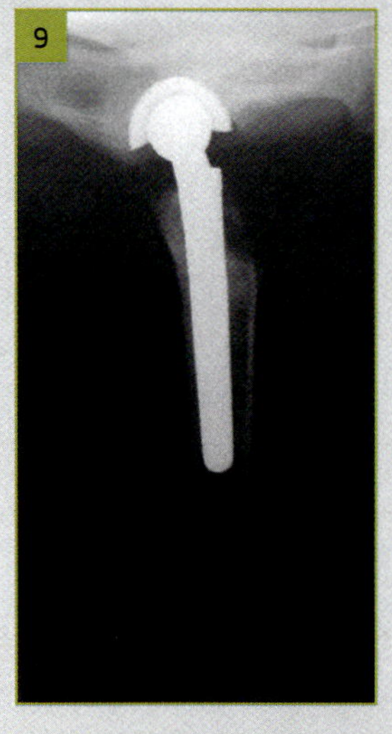

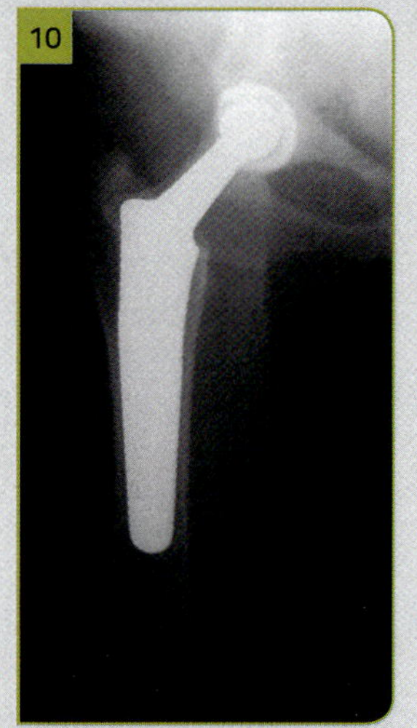

Figure 8. Ventrodorsal view of a prosthetic replacement arthroplasty.

Figure 9. Laterolateral view of a prosthetic replacement arthroplasty.

Figure 10. Craniocaudal view of a prosthetic replacement arthroplasty.

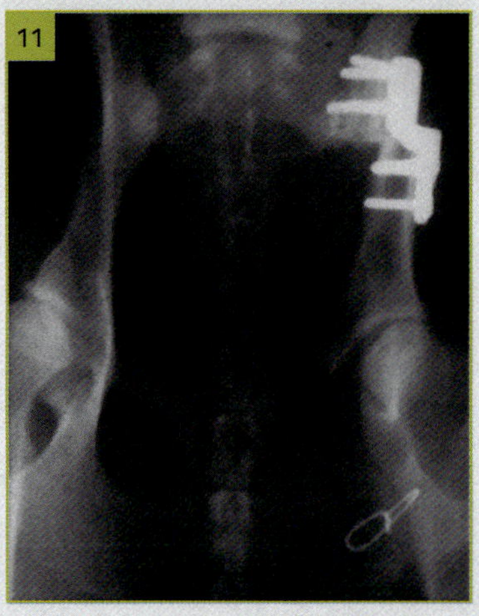

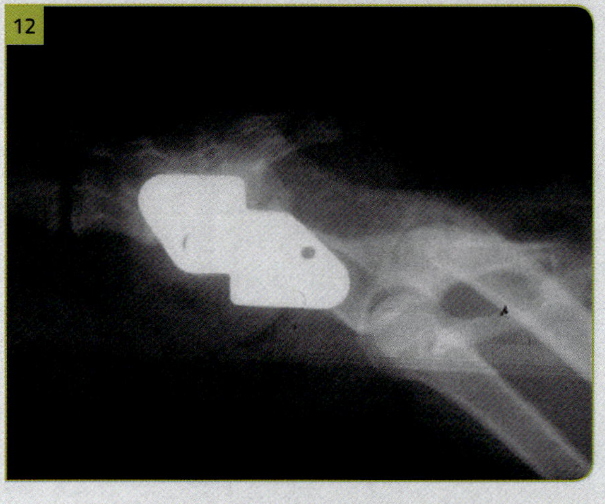

Figure 11. Ventrodorsal view of surgical correction of hip dysplasia using TPO (Triple Pelvic Osteotomy).

Figure 12. Laterolateral view of surgical correction of hip dysplasia using TPO.

Treatment

There are three key lines of treatment for hip dysplasia: classic (excision arthroplasty, pectinectomy and/or medical treatment), prosthetic or replacement arthroplasty (Figs. 8, 9 and 10) and osteotomy (Figs. 11 and 12).

There are three different types of osteotomy:

- **Pelvic osteotomy:** the purpose of this procedure is to rotate the acetabulum to improve coverage of the femoral head by the dorsal acetabular rim, obviously because there is insufficient coverage (acetabular hyperinclination) and subluxation. The ultimate goal is to reposition the acetabulum into a more favourable and biomechanical position; a congruent position, i.e. with an optimum fit between the two surfaces of the joint, and a stable position, i.e. the capacity for one joint surface to remain inside the other.
- **Femoral head osteotomy:** this procedure is indicated for cases of coxa valga, and can be performed in two ways (or a combination of the both):
  - **Femoral varisation osteotomy:** this technique involves placing the femoral head in a more favourable biomechanical position, reducing the angle of inclination (varus).
  - **Femoral derotation osteotomy:** this procedure corrects excessively anteversive angles of inclination.

In adult animals weighing over 10-15 kg, presenting joint pain and instability but no degenerative changes, treatment consists of a corrective osteotomy - either pelvic or femoral, depending on a range of parameters.

Pelvic osteotomy is indicated where the acetabulum is clearly affected, in which case the condition initially presents instability of the joint as the acetabulum gradually reaches a position of hyperinclination. As the joint moves, the femoral head loses contact with the acetabular joint surfaces, only touching the more peripheral areas, thus causing a extra load on these areas. This overload causes inflammation of the cartilage and the subchondral bone, both in the acetabulum and the femoral head, thus causing pain. Over time, the condition is aggravated, thus increasing instability, acetabular hyperinclination and inflammation of the cartilage and subchondral bone. This evolves into subchondral sclerosis, and the acetabulum becomes worn down, causing a degenerative joint condition.

TPO is always indicated before these degenerative changes become evident (Figs. 13, 14 and 15). Where early diagnosis is not possible, palliative treatment is indicated, via pectineal tenotomy or a definitive solution with excision arthroplasty or hip replacement.

It should be remembered that the ultimate purpose of TPO is to reposition the hyperinclined acetabulum into a correct position with normal inclination. This allows the acetabulum to provide more coverage for the femoral head and thus resolves the instability of the joint.

13

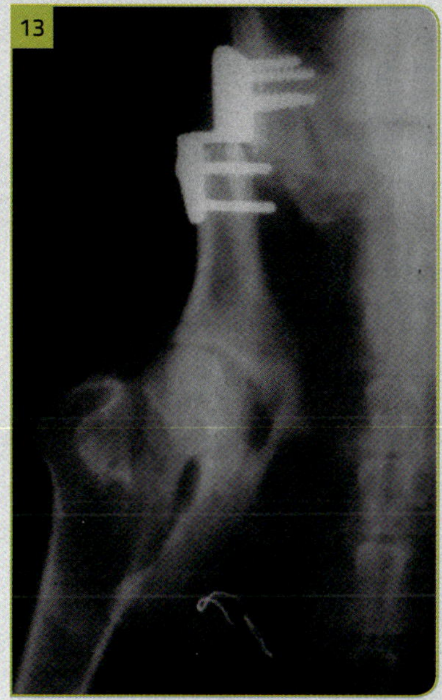

14

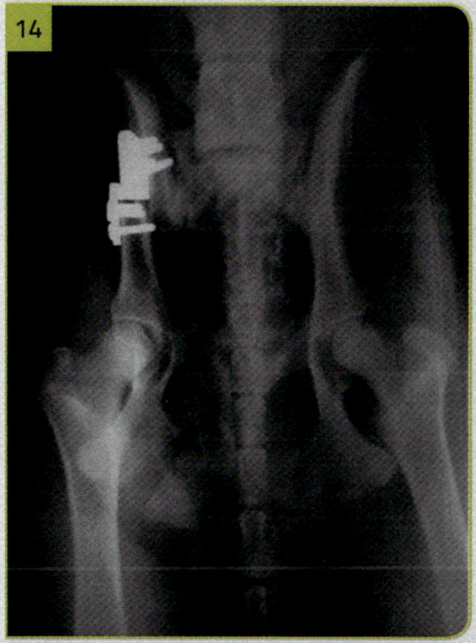

15

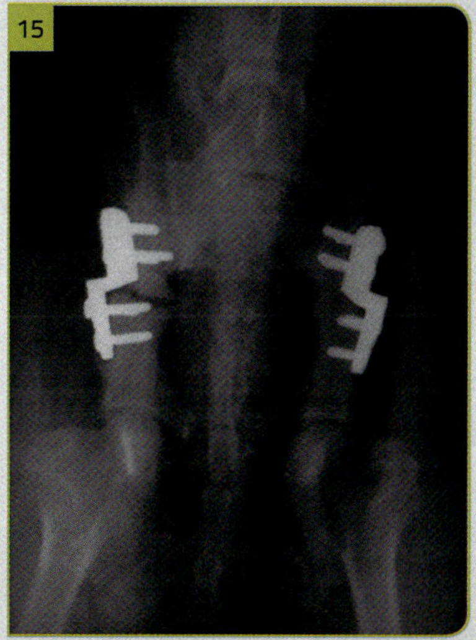

Figure 13. Hip dysplasia corrected using TPO surgery.

Figure 14. Ventrodorsal view of both hips after TPO.

Figure 15. Bilateral TPO.

02

Avascular necrosis of the femoral head

The atiopathogenesis of avascular necrosis of the femoral head, or Legg-Calvé-Perthes disease, is complex, and still the subject of many clinical and experimental studies.

In a single generation, there appear to be two main types of influencing factors; local factors and those depending on the constitution of the animal in question. Local factors in turn include both vascular and those inherent to tissue disorder.

It has been suggested that this necrosis is of ischemic origin, probably given the x-ray images of densification and collapse observed in this condition. This theory is supported by data such as the presence of necrotic laminar bone covered by immature bone tissue, sometimes viable and at other times also necrotic, and an increase in cervical pressure with alterations in the venous drainage pattern and diaphyseal fill.

Experiments have also demonstrated that in order to re-create this histological condition, the blood supply needs to be repeatedly interrupted. Furthermore, studies of the epiphyseal and cervical vasculature show that, despite the abundant circulation in young dogs, the blood supply to the ossification nucleus of the femoral head primarily depends on the ascending lateral or epiphyseal vessels and that the vessels do not penetrate the physis, but supply the area through the perichondral ring complex. In short, both the location and distribution of the epiphyseal vasculature are crucial.

The mechanism of vascular interruption is subject to debate, as no conclusive data has yet been obtained. Other authors suggest a concomitant tissue disorder, using the possible connection with transitory synovitis to propose a mechanism of intra-articular blockage. This means that the inflammation and effusion in the joint cause increases intracapsular pressure thus reducing flow through the small blood vessels, and triggering a mechanism similar to that observed in compartment syndrome. Furthermore, the frequency of trauma history and occurrence predominantly in generally more active male dogs would seem to suggest a connection between overloading of the joint and poor blood supply.

Recent studies have once again examined the connection between synovitis and perfusion defect. However, it must be remembered that, both at experimental and clinical level, it is difficult to establish whether the findings to which the cause of the condition is attributed appear prior to, or during (and therefore as a result of) the process.

Some of the observations made in the chondral areas underlying the joint cartilage of the affected femoral head have also been seen in the acetabulum and greater trochanter. A connection has also been suggested with other epiphyseal disorders in the form of irregularities of the ossification nucleus or full epiphysiolisis observed under X-ray.

As regards constitutional factors, numerous observations also confirm the presence of general physical characteristics in dogs with this condition in comparison to unaffected animals. It is well known that this condition is more common in certain breeds, in particular miniature or toy puppies. These small puppies are more susceptible to suffering from the condition, which is uncommon in large breeds. This explains why toy breed puppies, such as the Maltese or the Yorkshire Terrier, are particularly prone to lameness of this type, as biometrically they have shorter physical dimensions, especially in the distal region, although not so in the head or spine. Some hormonal alterations have also been observed, in particular somatomedins.

Diagnosis

Pain is mild to moderate and tends to appear when exercising, thus explaining the delay in consulting a veterinary clinic in many cases. Under examination, limited internal rotation and abduction is observed. The latter may be caused by contraction of the abductor muscles, or in severe and advanced cases, by femoral head deformity. Where there is muscular atrophy of the gluteal and quadriceps muscles it can be assumed that the condition has been present for some time.

In this condition, laboratory tests are negative, and are used to rule out other processes such as arthritis or osteomyelitis.

Craniocaudal and laterolateral X-ray projections show the images described above, and therefore help to rule out other conditions and confirm the diagnosis (Fig. 16).

Differential diagnosis

We recommend differential diagnosis, primarily with inflammatory conditions, which present greater intensity of pain, muscle contraction and limitation of movement, in addition to clinical and analytical systemic signs (leukocytosis, increased erythrocyte sedimentation rate -ESR-, etc.).

Treatment

Over the years, treatment for this condition has passed through successive cycles of abstention, conservative treatment and optimistic surgery. There is still no long term prospective study using consistent and stratified treatment based on age, gender, breed, etc.

Having established the inefficacy and inconsistency of procedures based on taking weight off the joint, and having proven this to be impossible in practice, the concept of epiphyseal containment emerged. According to this theory, the placing of the entire epiphyseal nucleus within the confines of the acetabulum during the fragmentation phase would provide adequate protection and a morphological mould for the joint to heal away from deforming mechanical factors, predominantly in the dorsolateral region.

The ideal position is achieved with the hip joint in abduction and internally rotated, using conservative procedures (strapping) or surgery (femoral varisation osteotomy or TPO).

Orthopaedic abduction devices present certain disadvantages making them difficult to use given the size of the animals in question.

Intertrochanteric varisation and derotation osteotomy aligns the distal part of the limb with the axis of the body, keeping the proximal end of the femur in the desired position; however, this procedure is highly complex. TPO is more appropriate, however any failure requires two surgical procedures, each with its corresponding cost. The consolidation of the joint is ensured by fixing a a plate, although this is difficult to implement given the small size of the animals in question.

Where the femoral head cannot be contained or the animal is in the healing stage, the prognosis is poor, and the above surgical options are less effective. In clinical practice these cases are treated with excision arthroplasty (Figs. 17 and 18).

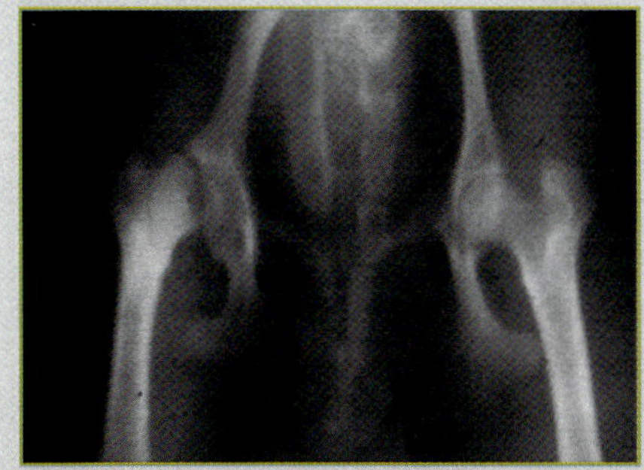

Figure 16. Diagnostic image, together with clinical data and type of animal.

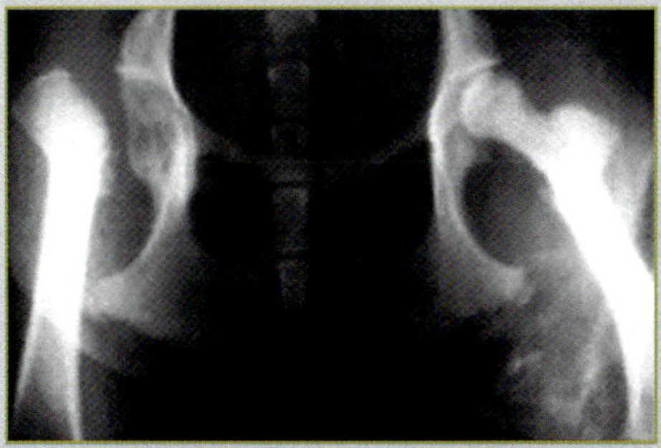

Figure 17. Surgical treatment using excision arthroplasty.

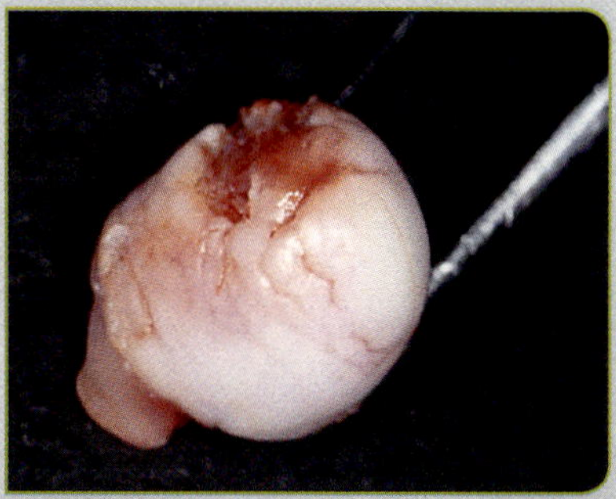

Figure 18. Detailed view of femoral head after surgical removal.

Diagnostic imaging techniques

The following are pairs of images showing transparent plastinated sections of real structures compared with images obtained using CAT and MRI.

Transparent plastinated sections + CAT

HORIZONTAL SECTION OF THE COXOFEMORAL JOINT AT MAXIMUM EXTENSION

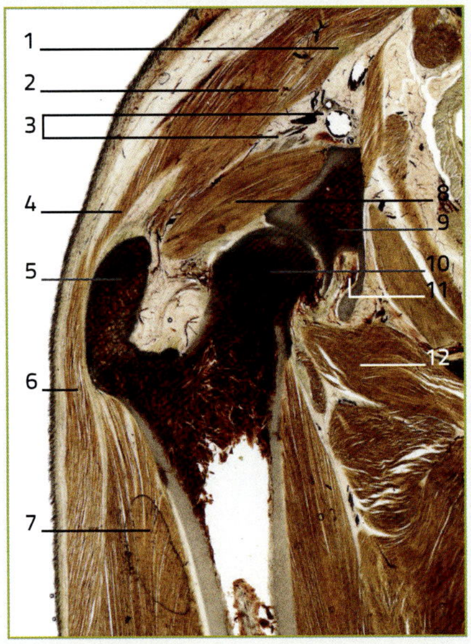

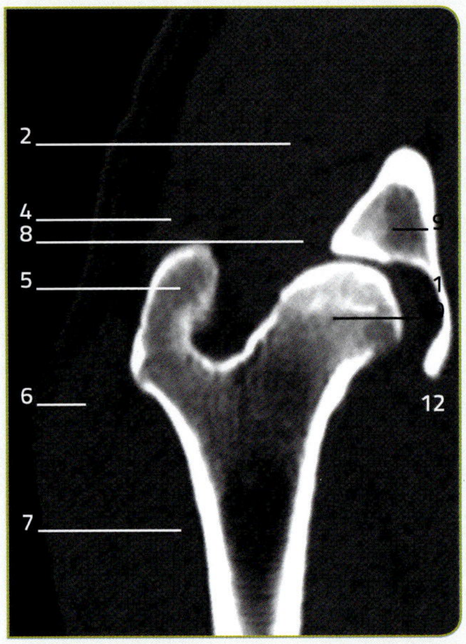

1	Sacrotuberous lig.
2	Middle gluteal muscle
3	Sciatic nerve, caudal gluteal artery and vein
4	Superficial gluteal muscle
5	Greater trochanter
6	Biceps femoris muscle
7	Quadriceps femoris muscle
8	Deep gluteal muscle
9	Acetabulum
10	Femoral head
11	Femoral head lig.
12	Iliopsoas muscle

TRANSVERSAL SECTION OF THE COXOFEMORAL JOINT AT MAXIMUM EXTENSION

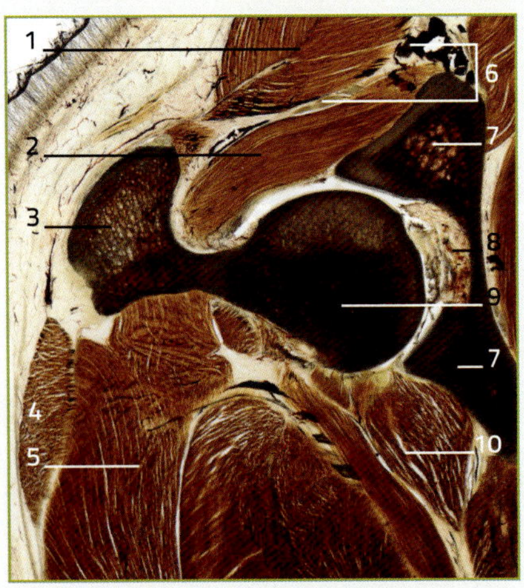

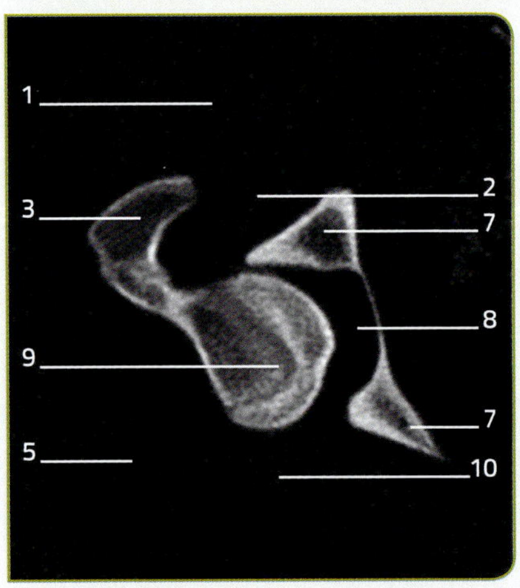

1	Middle gluteal muscle
2	Gemelli muscles
3	Greater trochanter
4	Tensor fascia latae muscle
5	Quadriceps femoris muscle
6	Sciatic nerve, caudal gluteal artery and vein
7	Acetabulum
8	Femoral head lig.
9	Femoral head
10	Iliopsoas muscle

Transparent plastinated sections + MRI

HORIZONTAL SECTION OF THE COXOFEMORAL JOINT AT MAXIMUM EXTENSION

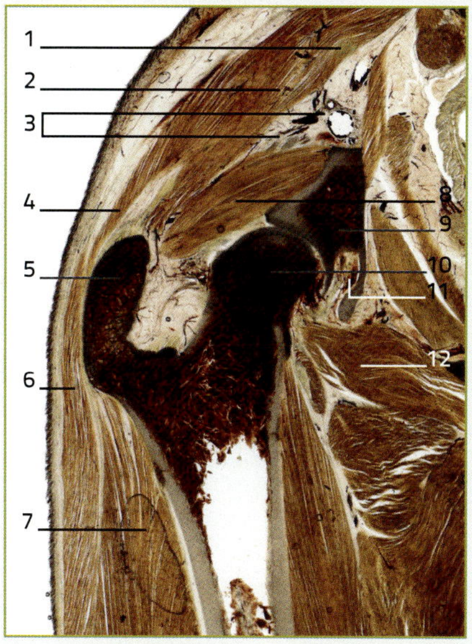

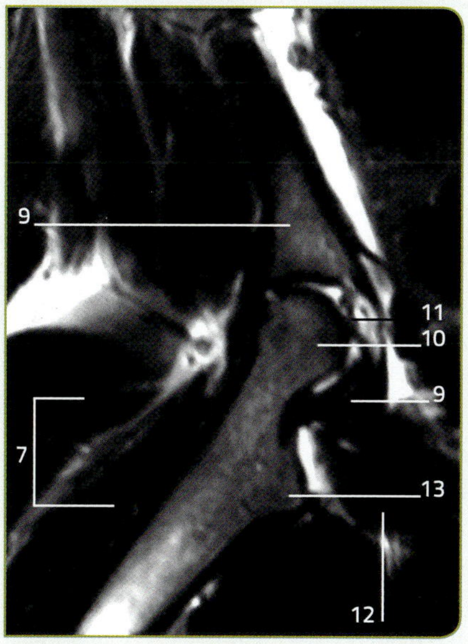

1	Sacrotuberous lig.
2	Middle gluteal muscle
3	Sciatic nerve, caudal gluteal artery and vein
4	Superficial gluteal muscle
5	Greater trochanter
6	Biceps femoris muscle
7	Quadriceps femoris muscle
8	Deep gluteal muscle
9	Acetabulum
10	Femoral head
11	Femoral head lig.
12	Iliopsoas muscle
13	Lesser trochanter

TRANSVERSAL SECTION OF THE COXOFEMORAL JOINT AT MAXIMUM EXTENSION

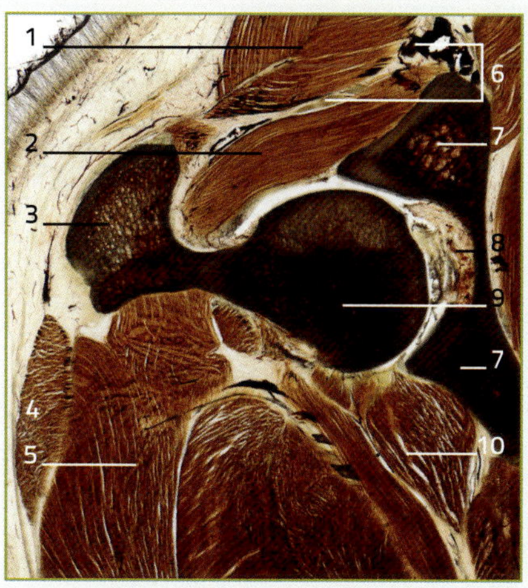

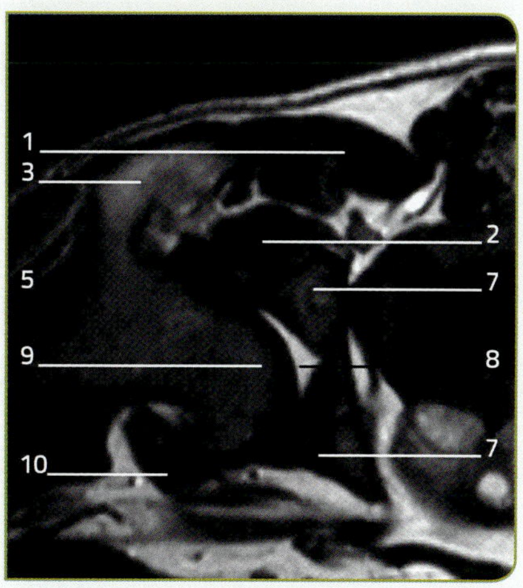

1	Middle gluteal muscle
2	Gemelli muscles
3	Greater trochanter
4	Tensor fascia latae muscle
5	Quadriceps femoris muscle
6	Sciatic nerve, caudal gluteal artery and vein
7	Acetabulum
8	Femoral head lig.
9	Femoral head
10	Iliopsoas muscle

SURGICAL APPROACHES

Craniodorsal approach to the hip joint via craniolateral incision

1 The skin incision is made taking the greater trochanter of the femur as a reference point, running towards the iliac crest and the middle third of the femur.

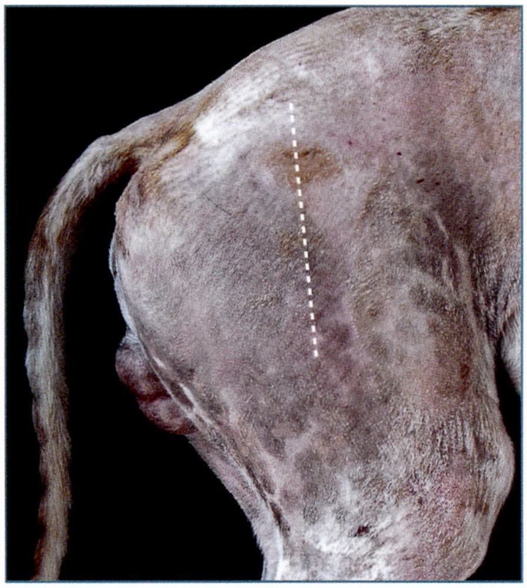

2 After resection of the gluteal fascia, the space between the middle gluteal muscle and the tensor fascia latae muscle is identified.

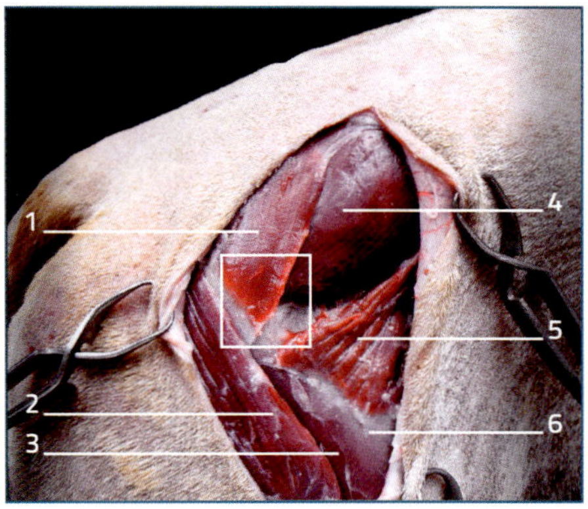

1 Superficial gluteal muscle
2 Biceps femoris muscle
3 Vastus lateralis muscle
4 Middle gluteal muscle
5 Tensor fascia latae muscle
6 Fascia lata

3 Enlargement of the previous image. The space between the middle gluteal muscle and the tensor fascia latae muscle is identified, permitting a cranial approach to the hip joint.

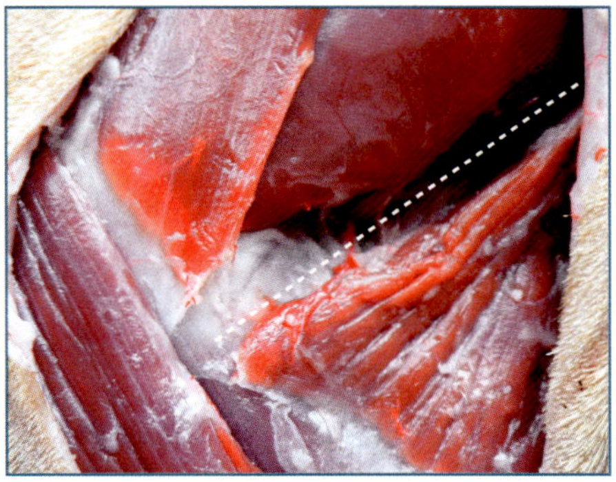

4 By displacing the middle gluteal muscle dorsally and the tensor fascia latae muscle ventrally the space between the deep gluteal, rectus femoris and vastus lateralis muscles can be located for access to the joint itself. Care must be taken not to damage the cranial gluteal nerve.

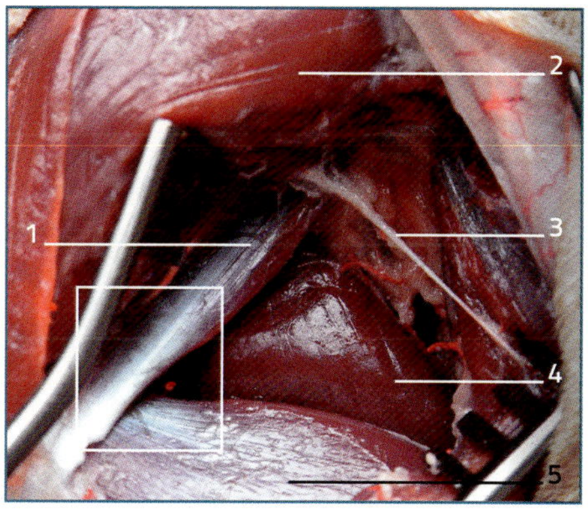

1 Deep gluteal muscle
2 Middle gluteal muscle
3 Cranial gluteal nerve
4 Rectus femoris muscle
5 Vastus lateralis muscle

5 After placing the separator into the intermuscular space described above, the articular capsule is exposed, covered by the articular muscle of the hip joint.

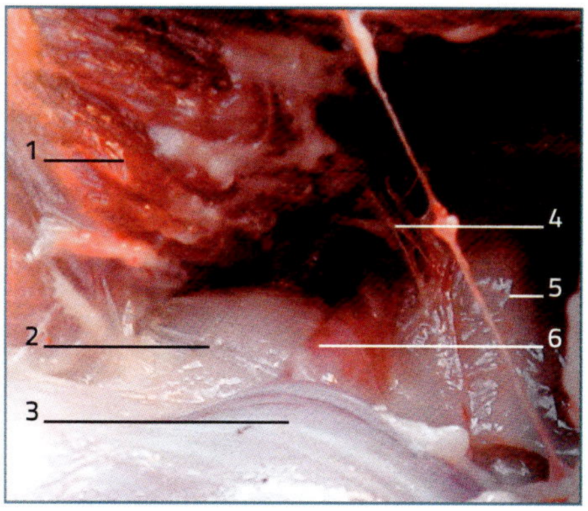

1 Deep gluteal muscle
2 Articular capsule
3 Vastus lateralis muscle
4 Muscular branches of the lateral circumflex femoral vessels
5 Rectus femoris muscle
6 Articular muscle of the hip joint

6 By sectioning the articular capsule the femoral head can be examined. The joint can be further exposed by partial tenotomy of the deep gluteal muscle and by external femoral rotation.

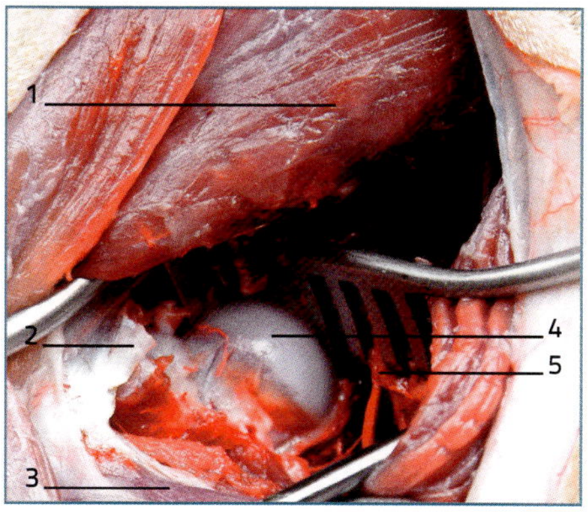

1 Middle gluteal muscle
2 Deep gluteal muscle tendon
3 Vastus lateralis muscle
4 Femoral head
5 Muscular branches of the lateral circumflex femoral vessels

Craniodorsal and caudodorsal approach to the hip joint via osteotomy of the greater trochanter

1 The skin incision is made taking the greater trochanter as a reference point, extending proximally towards the iliac crest and distally towards the femur. After resection of the gluteal fascia, the meeting point between the biceps femoris and superficial gluteal muscles is identified.

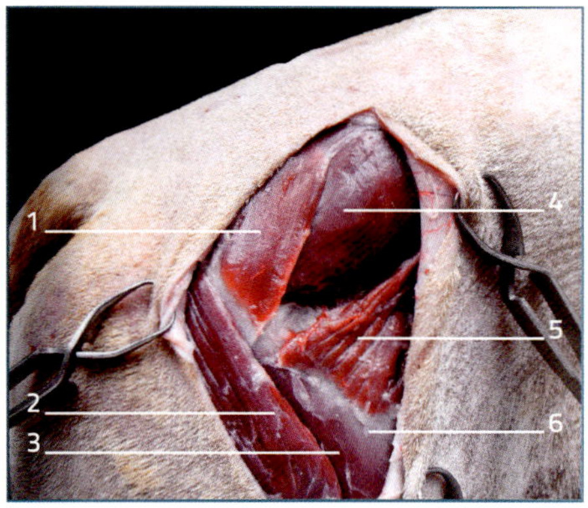

1 Superficial gluteal muscle
2 Biceps femoris muscle
3 Vastus lateralis muscle
4 Middle gluteal muscle
5 Tensor fascia latae muscle
6 Fascia lata

2 After osteotomy of the greater trochanter at an angle of 45° in a dorsomedial direction, it can be seen how the group of muscles with their point of insertion on the trochanter can also be displaced along with it.

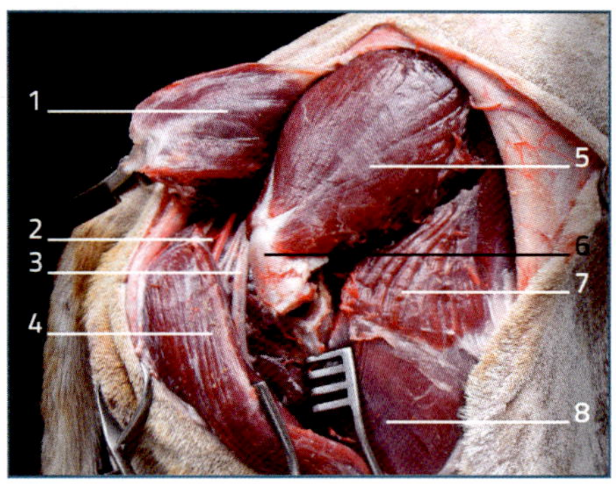

1 Superficial gluteal muscle
2 Caudal gluteal artery and vein
3 Sciatic nerve
4 Biceps femoris muscle
5 Middle gluteal muscle
6 Greater trochanter
7 Tensor fascia latae muscle
8 Vastus lateralis muscle

3 The greater trochanter and the middle and deep gluteal muscles, together with the piriform muscle, have been displaced dorsally. After sectioning the articular capsule access to the femoral head is obtained. The joint surfaces can be further exposed by forcing adduction of the femur. The proximity of the sciatic nerve and the caudal gluteal blood vessels to the line of the osteotomy can be observed.

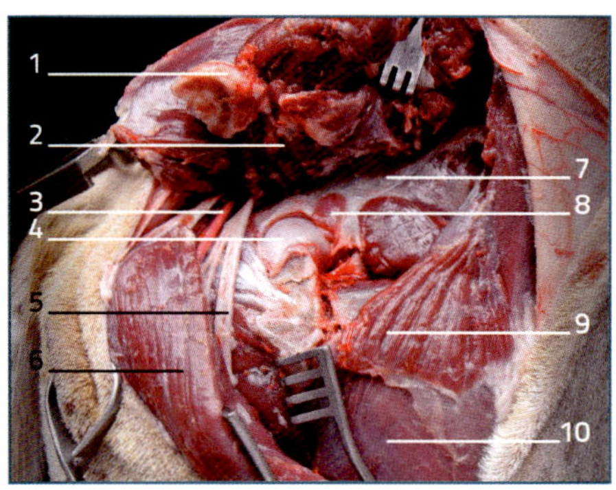

1 Greater trochanter
2 Gluteal muscles
3 Caudal gluteal artery and vein
4 Femoral head
5 Sciatic nerve
6 Biceps femoris muscle
7 Wing of ilium
8 Articular muscle of the hip joint
9 Tensor fascia latae muscle
10 Vastus lateralis muscle

4 Dorsal displacement of the origin of the middle gluteal muscle exposes the wing of ilium.

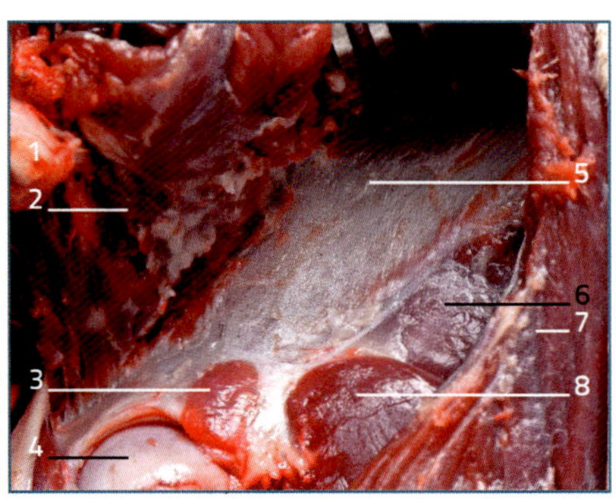

1 Greater trochanter
2 Gluteal muscles
3 Articular muscle of the hip joint
4 Femoral head
5 Wing of ilium
6 Iliac muscle
7 Tensor fascia latae muscle
8 Rectus femoris muscle

5 The central or acetabular portion of the hip bone can be observed upon dorsal displacement of the greater trochanter and the gluteal muscles.

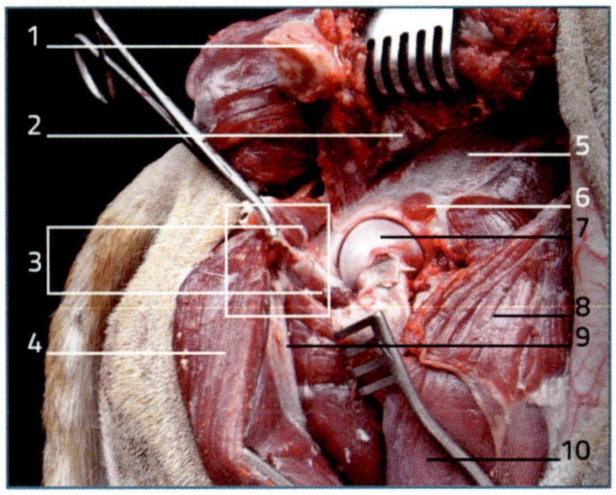

1 Greater trochanter
2 Gluteal muscles
3 Gemelli and internal obturator muscles
4 Biceps femoris muscle
5 Wing of ilium
6 Articular muscle of the hip joint
7 Femoral head
8 Tensor fascia latae muscle
9 Sciatic nerve
10 Vastus lateralis muscle

6 In order to access the caudal portion of the hip bone, the insertions of the gemelli and internal obturator muscles must be sectioned.

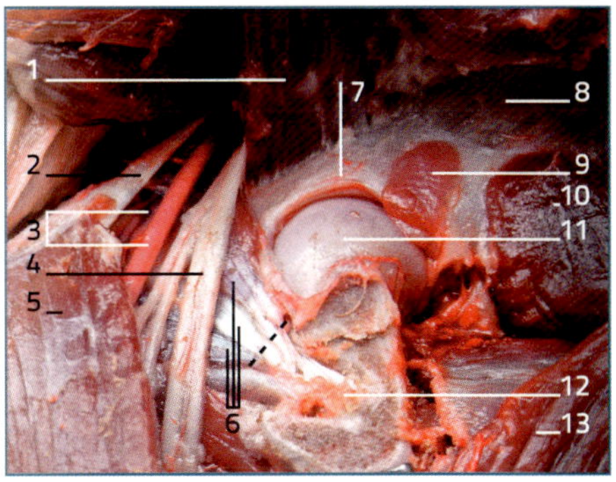

1 Gluteal muscles
2 Sacrotuberous ligament
3 Caudal gluteal artery and vein
4 Sciatic nerve
5 Biceps femoris muscle
6 Gemelli and internal obturator muscles
7 Dorsal acetabular rim
8 Wing of ilium
9 Articular muscle of the hip joint
10 Rectus femoris muscle
11 Femoral head
12 Trochanteric fossa
13 Tensor fascia latae muscle

7 After completing the tenotomy of the gemelli and internal obturator muscles, they are retracted dorsally, exposing the caudal acetabular rim and part of the body of ischium, without the need for sectioning the insertion of the external obturator muscle.

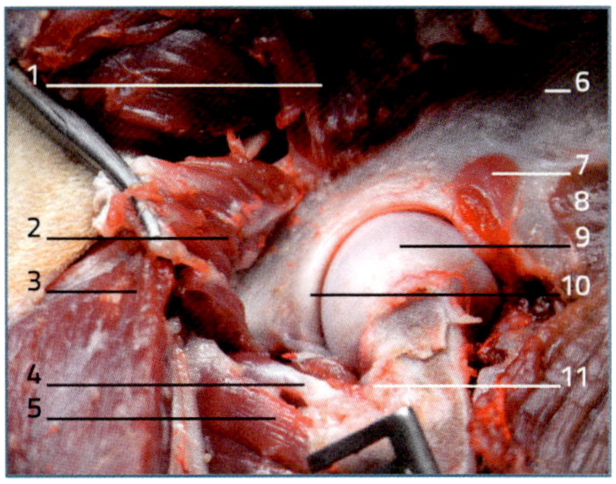

1 Gluteal muscles
2 Gemelli and internal obturator muscles
3 Biceps femoris muscle
4 Tendon of the external obturator muscle
5 Quadratus femoris muscle
6 Wing of ilium
7 Articular muscle of the hip joint
8 Rectus femoris muscle
9 Femoral head
10 Caudal acetabular rim
11 Trochanteric fossa

Craniodorsal and caudodorsal approach to the hip joint via tenotomy of the gluteal muscles

1 It can be seen how the middle and deep gluteal muscles have been detached and displaced dorsally, together with the piriform muscle. After sectioning the articular capsule and forcing external femoral rotation, the femoral head is exposed.

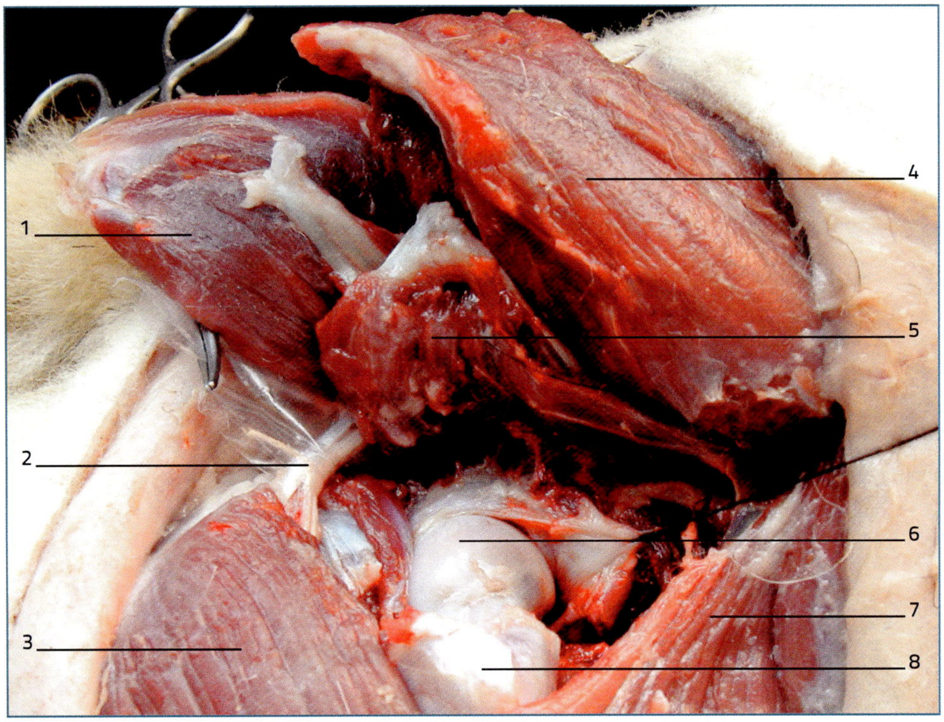

1 Superficial gluteal muscle
2 Sciatic nerve and caudal gluteal artery and vein
3 Biceps femoris muscle
4 Middle gluteal muscle
5 Deep gluteal muscle
6 Femoral head
7 Tensor fascia latae muscle
8 Greater trochanter

Ventral approach to hip joint and pubis

1 The animal is placed in lateral recumbency with abducted contralateral limb. The skin incision is made over the shape of the pectineus muscle.

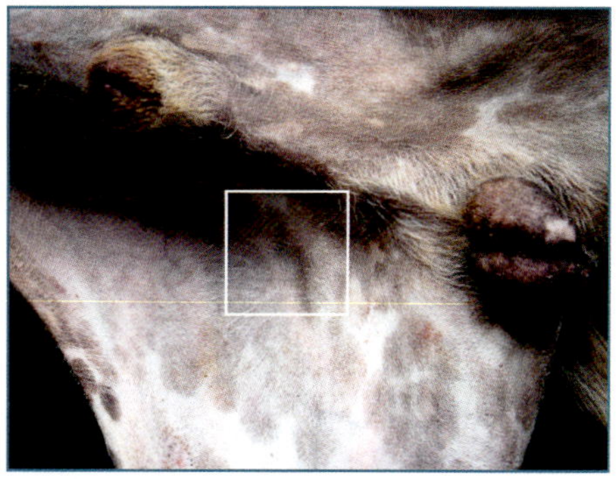

2 After sectioning the fascia, the femoral artery and vein are located, running through the femoral canal between the pectineus and sartorius muscles. To access the ventral surface of the hip joint the origin of the pectineus muscle at the pubis must be sectioned.

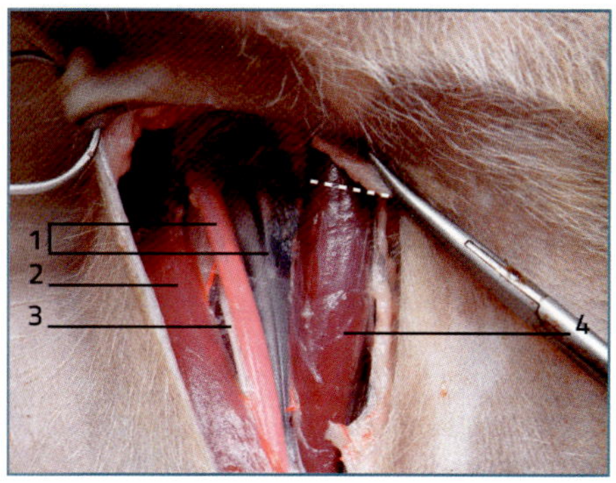

1 Femoral artery and vein
2 Sartorius muscle, caudal portion
3 Saphenous nerve
4 Pectineus muscle

3 The femoral head is exposed by displacing the pectineus muscle ventrally and sectioning the articular capsule. The iliopsoas muscle has been displaced ventrally and the medial circumflex femoral artery has been moved dorsally.

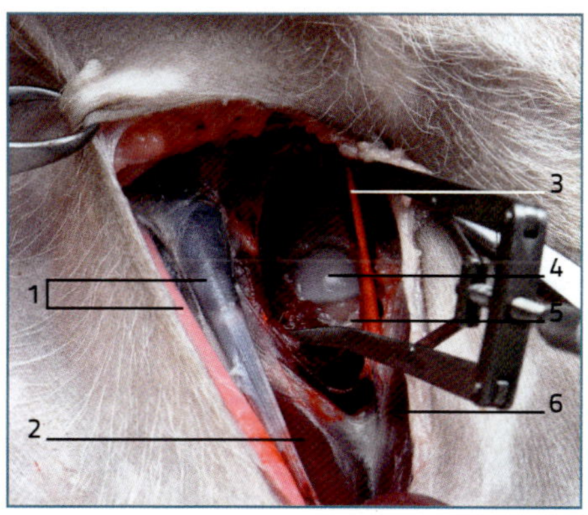

1 Femoral artery and vein
2 Sartorius muscle, caudal portion
3 Medial circumflex femoral artery
4 Femoral head
5 Articular capsule
6 Pectineus muscle

4 The medial circumflex femoral artery can be displaced ventrally in order to expose the ventral acetabular rim and the body of the pubic bone more easily. Forcing the abduction of the femur facilitates further exposure of the femoral head.

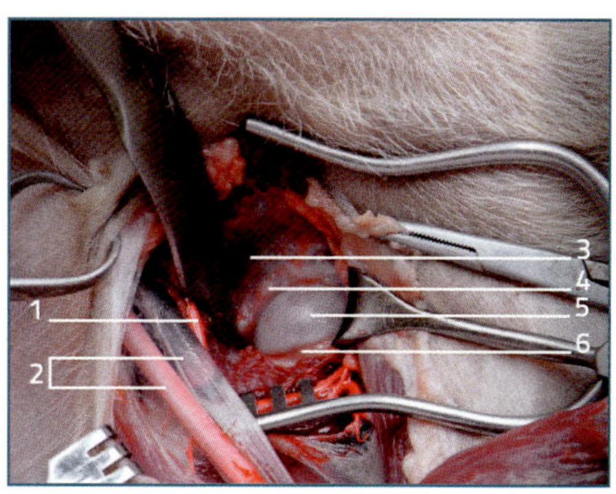

1 Medial circumflex femoral artery
2 Femoral artery and vein
3 Pubic bone
4 Acetabulum, ventral rim
5 Femoral head
6 Articular capsule

The images included for surgical approaches are adapted from: Latorre, R., Gil, F., Climent, S., López, O., Henry, R., Ayala, M., Ramírez, G., Martínez, F., Vázquez, J.M. *Color Atlas of Surgical Approaches to the Bones and Joints of the Dog and Cat*. Intermédica S.A., 2009; pp. 0-266. ISBN 978-950-555-353-2.

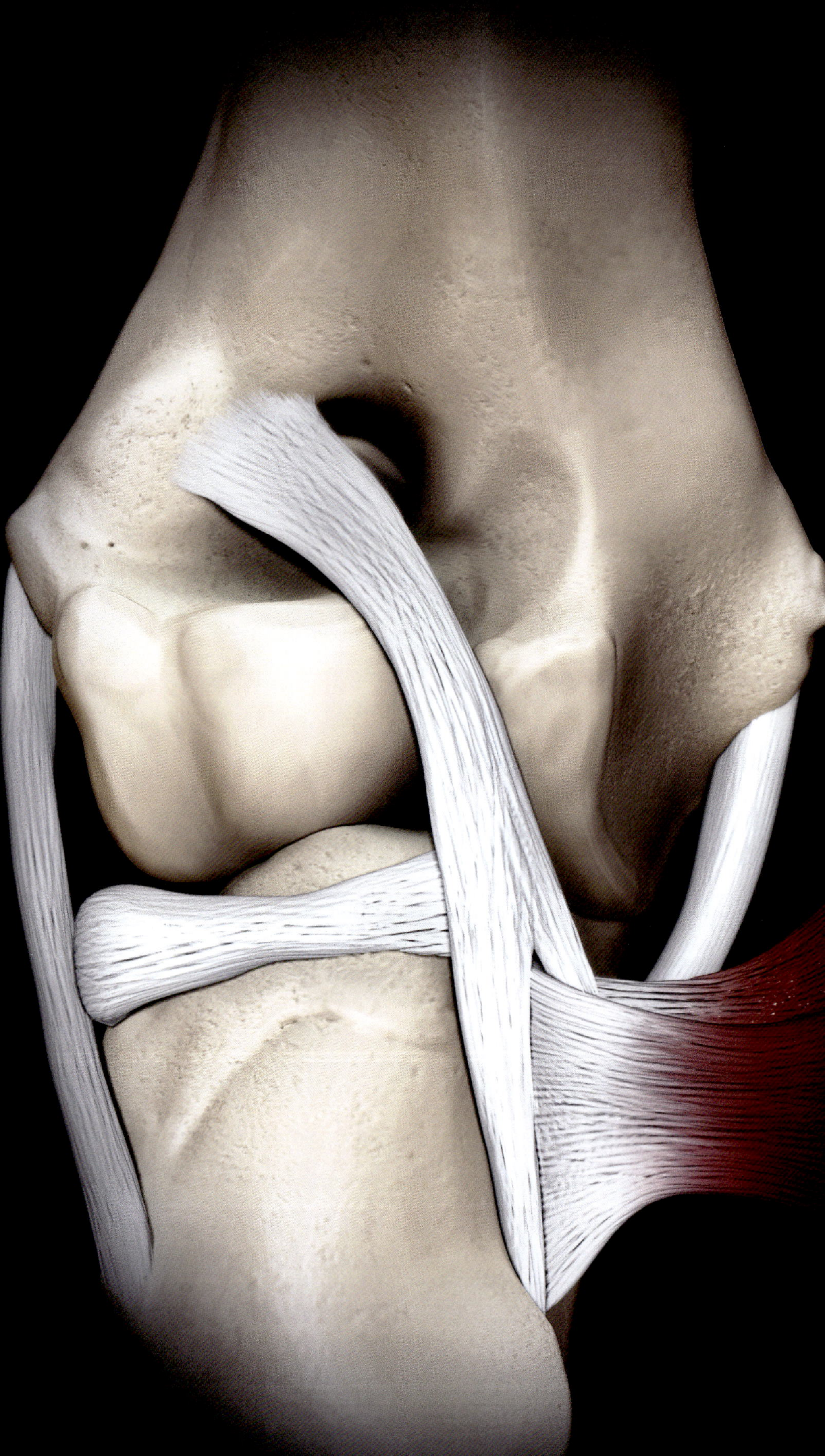

ELBOW JOINT

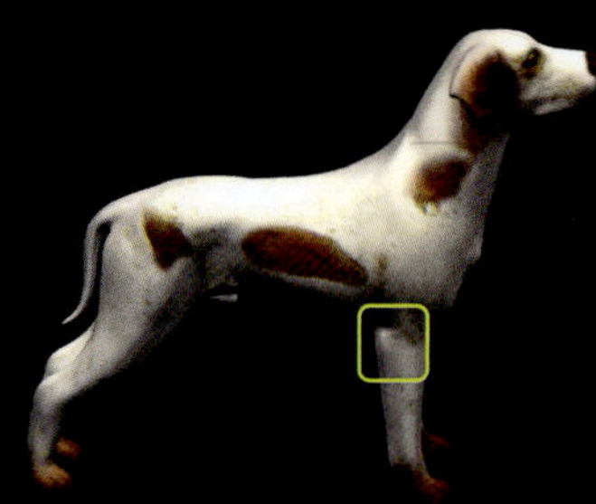

Elbow joint

Watch this video on the electronic version
Thoracic limb

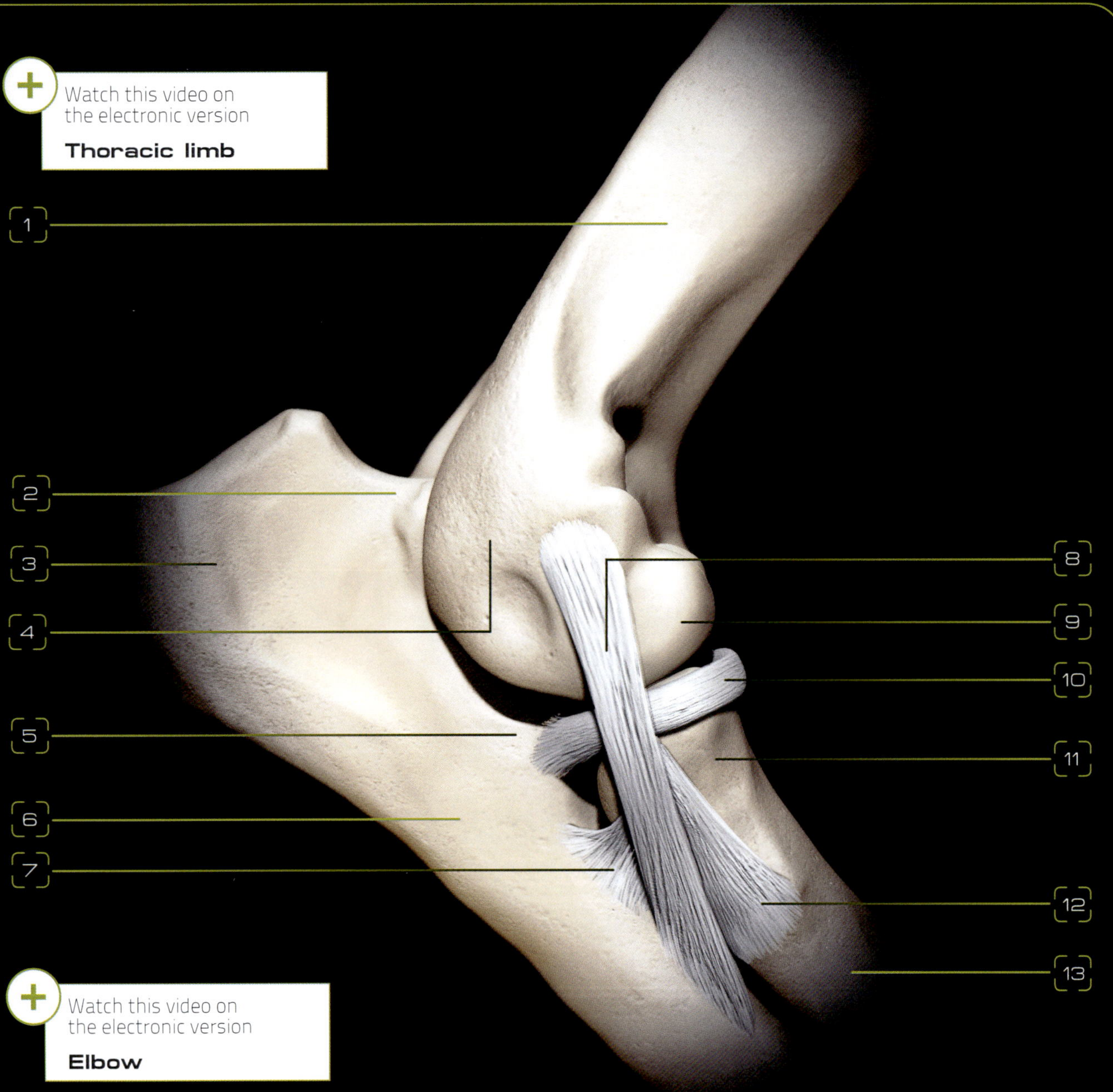

Watch this video on the electronic version
Elbow

LATERAL VIEW

1 Humerus
2 Anconeal apophysis
3 Olecranon
4 Lateral epicondyle of the humerus
5 Lateral coronoid apophysis
6 Ulna
7 Lateral collateral lig., caudal part
8 Lateral collateral lig.
9 Condyle of the humerus, capitulum
10 Annular lig.
11 Head of radius
12 Lateral collateral lig., cranial part
13 Radius

CRANIAL VIEW

1 Supratrochlear foramen
2 Lateral epicondyle of the humerus
3 Condyle of the humerus, capitulum
4 Lateral collateral lig.
5 Annular lig.
6 Head of radius
7 Oblique lig.
8 Medial epicondyle of the humerus
9 Medial collateral lig.
10 Biceps brachii muscle
11 Fibrous sheath supporting oblique lig.
12 Tendon of the brachial muscle

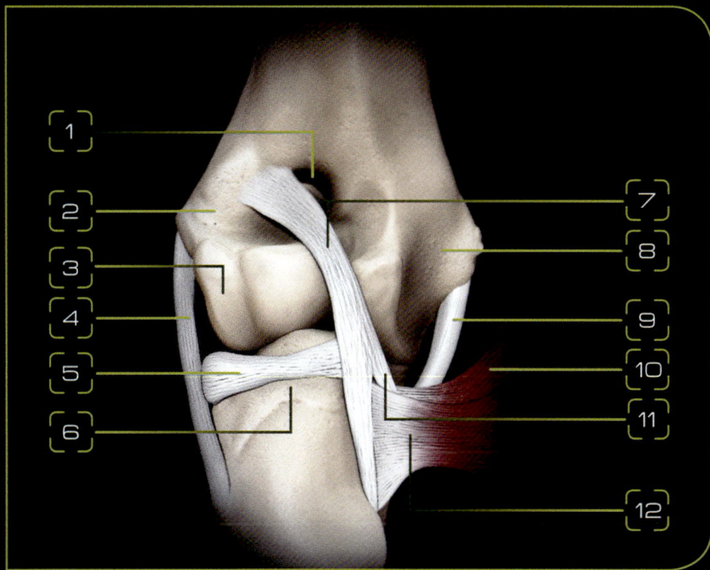

MEDIAL VIEW

1 Medial epicondyle of the humerus
2 Medial collateral lig.
3 Medial collateral lig., cranial part
4 Tendon of the brachial muscle
5 Fibrous sheath supporting oblique lig.
6 Tendon of the biceps brachii muscle
7 Ulna
8 Olecranon
9 Condyle of the humerus, trochlea
10 Medial coronoid apophysis
11 Medial collateral lig., caudal part

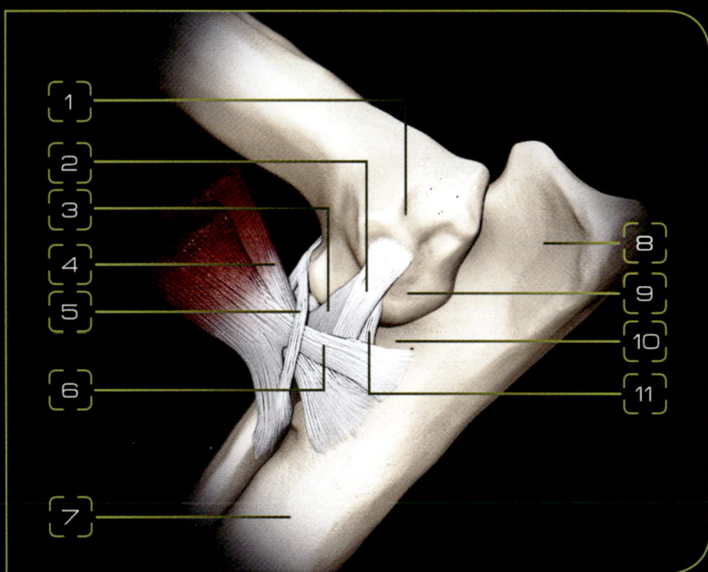

DORSOCAUDAL VIEW

1 Anconeal apophysis of the ulna
2 Olecranon fossa
3 Medial epicondyle of the humerus
4 Brachial muscle
5 Biceps brachii muscle
6 Medial collateral lig.
7 Olecranon
8 Olecranon tuberosity
9 Lateral epicondyle of the humerus
10 Olecranon lig.
11 Lateral collateral lig.

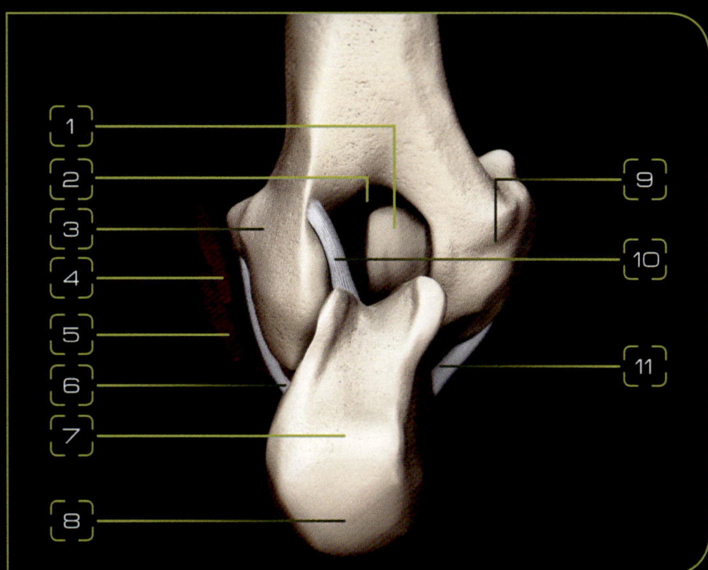

Orthopaedic conditions of the elbow

The term "elbow dysplasia" encompasses different forms of joint pathology, including:

01 Fragmented coronoid process (FCP)

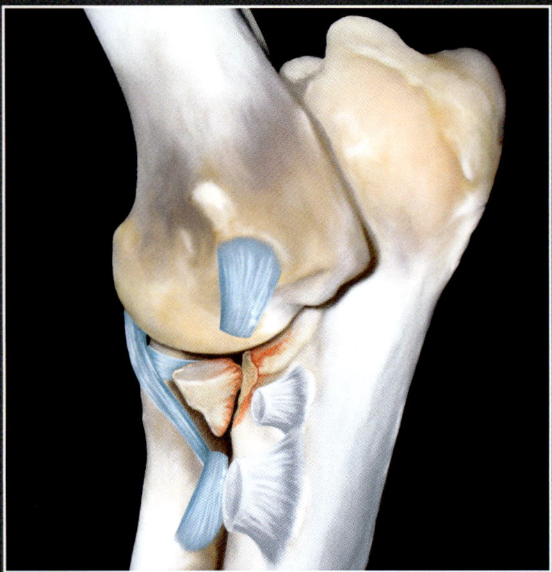

02 Osteochondrosis dissecans (OCD)

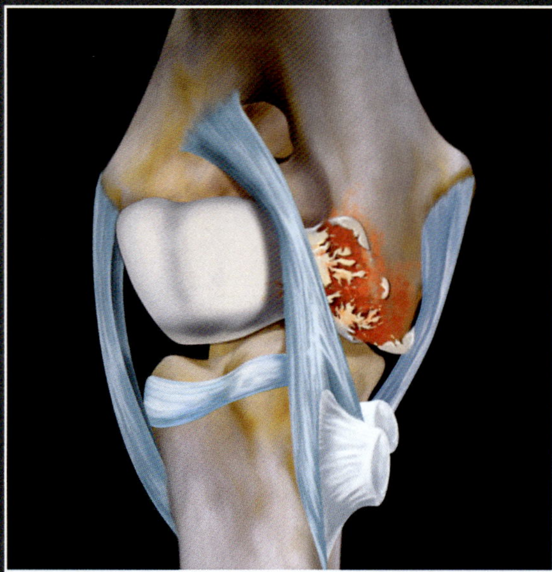

03 Ununited anconeal process (UAP)

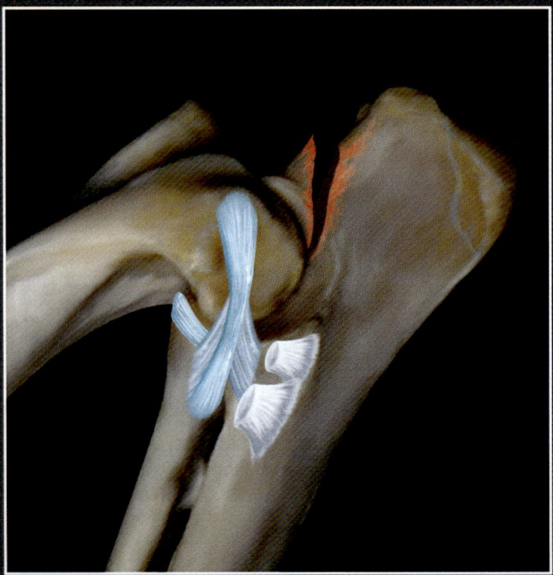

04 Joint incongruity (JI)

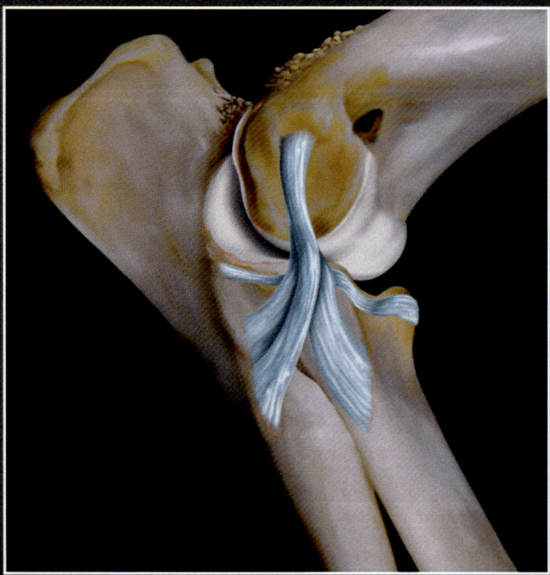

The joint between the humerus, radius and ulna constitutes one of the most complex in the body, as it is formed by three irregular surfaces of three different bones: firstly the condyles of the humerus, which develop from two different nuclei of ossification and later fuse with the diaphysis; the proximal epiphysis of the radius, with its nucleus of ossification and another in the distal area, which together determine the axial development of the bone; and finally, the ulna grows lengthways from the distal epiphysis and its formation in the joint is created by the proximal growth cartilage, thus completing the bone structure of the elbow joint. Any alteration in the growth rate of these points, either individually or collectively, results in the appearance of incongruity at the articular surfaces of the joint. In all cases these alterations affected the elbow joint in growing dogs, due to abnormalities in the nuclei of ossification, the development of one or more of the bones making up the joint, or a combination of both, resulting in articular incongruity. This condition presents in different forms of joint pathologies, known as: fragmented coronoid process (FCP); osteochondrosis dissecans (OCD), generally of the medial humeral condyle; ununited anconeal process (UAP); joint incongruity (JI); incomplete ossification of the humeral condyle and ununited medial epicondyle of the humerus (UME) (Fig. 1).

All these pathologies are grouped together under the term "elbow dysplasia" (ED). This term was originally coined by the International Working Elbow Group (IWEG) and initially adopted by other authors. It is currently in widespread use, although from a practical viewpoint it would be more correct to refer to "osteoarthritis of the elbow", although dysplasia is appropriate, given that osteoarthritis is a consequence of the condition.

Despite sharing common symptoms, these pathologies have not been proven to develop under similar ethologies; nor has any overlap of causal factors been observed. What has been confirmed is the genetic

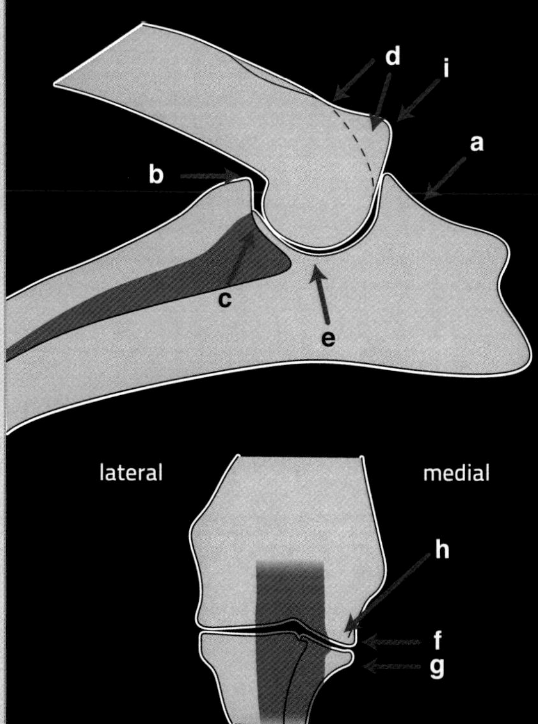

Figure 1. Diagram of the main points of diagnosis for elbow evaluation (IWEG).

a. Dorsal surface of anconeal process.
b. Cranial edge of the head of the radius.
c. Cranial margin of the medial coronoid process.
d. Caudal surface of the lateral epicondylar crest.
e. Ulnar sclerosis of the ulna at the trochlear notch.
f. Medial surface of medial epicondyle.
g. Medial edge of the medial coronoid process.
h. Identification point of subchondral bone.
i. Formation of osteophytes on the caudal edge of the medial epicondylar crest.

component of all these pathologies, and it has been suggested that inheritability may be specific to each clinical condition given the incident rate in each breed. Furthermore, key factors in the development of endochondral ossification, such as overfeeding with high phosphorous or high-protein diets or trauma incidents, must be taken into account when assessing ED. An incorrect size of the ulna and radius at the ulnar notch, thus not allowing the humeral trochlea to be housed properly, should be considered a common aetiology leading to FCP, OCD and UAP. Males are affected 75 % more frequently than bitches.

Given the frequency rate of these pathologies and the resulting disability, they have been the subject of a wide range of research, primarily by IWEG, which since 1989 has been devoted to clarifying all the aspects of these diseases and to the study of reproduction in different breeds through the formulation of assessment and control criteria, accepted worldwide today by both professionals and institutions such as the *Fédération Cynologique Internationale* (World Canine Organisation) and the World Small Animal Veterinary Association (WSAVA).

IWEG recommends using a scoring system for ED based on the level of osteophytes present in different areas of the elbow, as marked in Figure 1 (Table 1).

Table 1. Grading of elbow dysplasia by size of osteophytes (IWEG).

- **Grade 0:** no evidence of osteophytes.
- **Grade 1:** osteophytes <2 mm.
- **Grade 2:** osteophytes from 2 to 5 mm.
- **Grade 3:** osteophytes >5 mm.

This assessment method allows us to correlate the clinical signs of the condition with X-ray observations. It also helps to establish that the presence of grades 2 and 3 in puppies aged 1 year are indicative of ED.

The most commonly affected dogs are large breeds, including: Rottweiler, Labrador, Golden Retriever, German Shepherd, Bull Mastiff, Collie, St. Bernard, Chow Chow, Pyrenean Mountain Dog and Airedale Terrier. It has also been observed in some terriers and even in Pomeranians.

ED may present initially as osteochondrosis with a thickening of the cartilage in one area of the joint surface, causing OCD. Where this occurs in the nuclei of ossification, it causes FCP, UAP and JI.

FCP was first described in 1974. The most commonly affected breeds are: Labrador, Rottweiler, German Shepherd, Bull Mastiff, Chow Chow and some mongrels. Other breeds known to present the condition are the Beagle, Shetland Sheepdog and the Pomeranian. Males are more commonly affected than females. Detection of the condition via the usual X-ray projections is difficult, thus complicating diagnosis and the evolution of the osteoarthritic process; CAT scans should therefore always be used (Fig. 2). Diagnosis is often based on the observation of characteristic secondary joint abnormalities. This pathology can also occur concomitantly with UAP. The most appropriate treatment is arthrotomy of the elbow, followed by removal of the apophysis or coronoid process (with or without curettage).

OCD has been defined as a highly inheritable multi-factor condition, primarily affecting the Labrador, Bernese Mountain Dog, Rottweiler and German Shepherd, although it may occasionally be found in any heavier breed or in mongrels. It primarily affects the medial condyle of the humerus. It can be treated medically and surgically, with no significant difference in results and the evolution of the joint condition (Figs. 3 and 4).

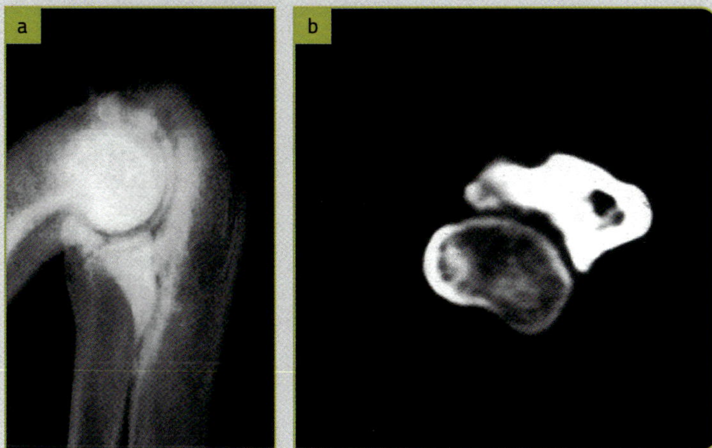

Figure 2. Fragmented coronoid process. Laterolateral X-ray (a) and CAT (b).

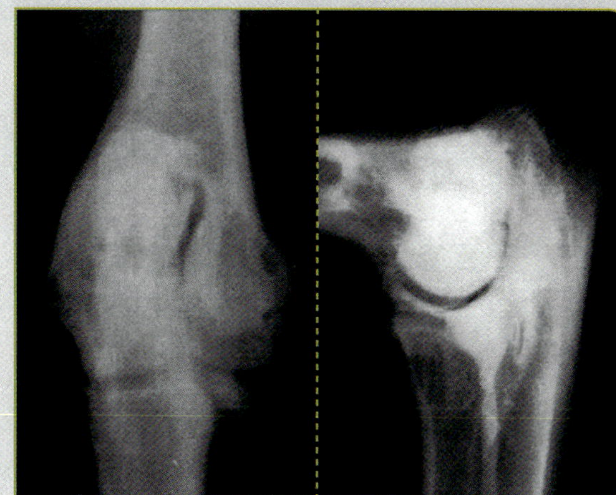

Figure 3. OCD; there is an alteration of the endochondral ossification process resulting in the separation of a portion of joint cartilage.

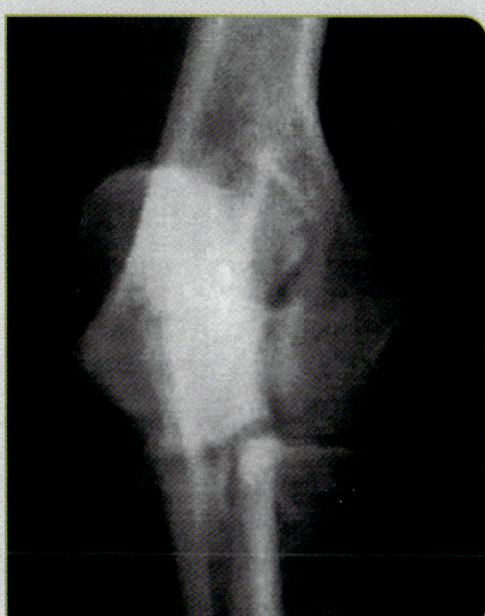

Figure 4. OCD; presence of a flap that remains attached.

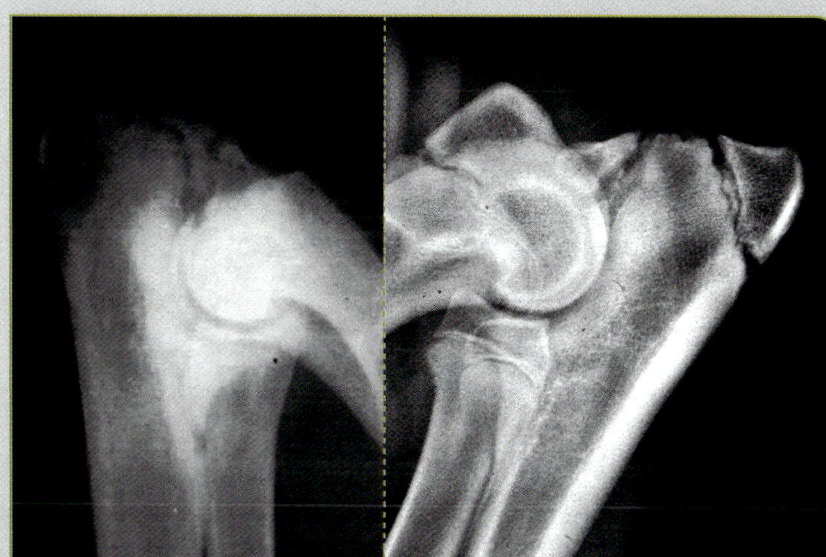

Figure 5. Ununited anconeal process.

UAP was first documented in 11 cases in German Shepherds. It is caused by a development issue in the nucleus of ossification. It is observed in chondrodystrophic breeds such as the Basset Hound and French Bulldog and in fast-growing non-chondrodystrophic breeds, most commonly affecting the German Shepherd. It has also been found in the St. Bernard, Great Dane, Labrador, Pointer and Pyrenean Mountain Dog. It frequently occurs concomitantly with other joint conditions, meaning that animals diagnosed with UAP must be examined closely in search of possible further abnormalities. The treatment of choice consists of early fixing, or removal, of the anconeal apophysis, in order to minimise the progress of degenerative joint disease (Fig. 5).

Despite the common clinical signs of these three pathologies, each also presents distinct characteristics to allow specific diagnosis. The implementation of palliative care during early study helps to delay the degenerative evolution of the condition.

JI may be the result of inherited anomalies, such as the presence of a sesamoid bone on the triceps tendon (patella cubiti), trauma, or premature closure of growth cartilage of the radius or ulna. Different surgical treatments are used for each case (Fig. 6).

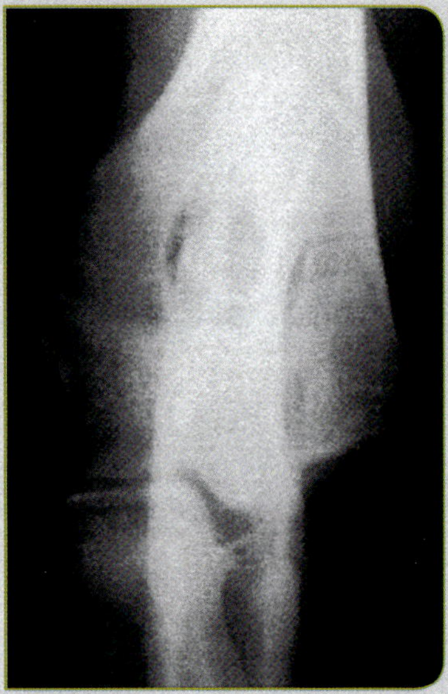

Figure 6. Joint incongruity; anatomical harmony has been lost as a result of growth abnormality.

These clinical cases present common symptoms. The onset of the condition occurs at an early age, between 4 and 7 months. Initially presents with intermittent and moderate claudication, becoming persistent and intense, with inflammation, effusion and a notable joint incongruity.

Susceptible breeds presenting an insidious claudication of the thoracic joint, together with the observation of some of the signs described above during clinical examination, should undergo detailed X-ray examinations. Early findings include joint effusion, fractures, wear or loss of cartilage in the trochlear notch, deformity of the anconeal apophysis, capsular thickening and the present of periarticular osteophytes (Fig. 7).

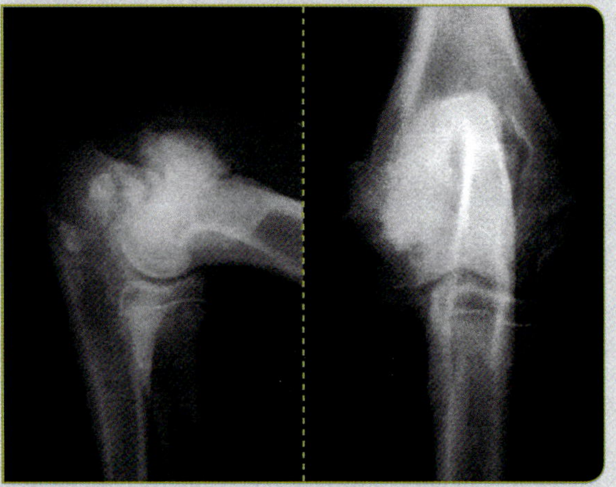

Figure 7. Severe osteoarthritis; osteophytes are observed in the trochlear notch and the medial condyle due to ununited medial humeral epicondyle (UME).

The individual diagnosis of each of the conditions involved in ED is complex; in the majority of cases due to the presence of common clinical signs and X-ray images, and also:

- Many clinical signs may go unnoticed due to the stoicism of the particular animal.
- In the habitual X-ray images of the elbow joint there is an overlapping of bone structures.
- The radiotransparency of the hyaline cartilage does not allow early detection of osteochondrosis.
- Two or more pathologies may occur simultaneously in the same joint.

Treatment of ED depends on the pathologies found. It is essential to commence treatment as soon as a firm diagnosis is obtained in order to limit osteoarthritic changes, which affect the degree of articular recovery.

Treatment can be conservative or surgical. The former is indicated only in cases presenting certain characteristics:

- Animals aged under 4-5 months, in which fusion of the anconeal process is not yet complete, but where it is seen to be correctly aligned and supported by fibrous tissue.
- Animals aged over 5 months, with very mild claudication and X-rays showing incipient osteoarthritic changes, without any evidence of coronoid fragmentation, OCD or UAP.
- Adult animals for which an accidental diagnosis of asymptomatic UAP or FCP is given.

Conservative treatment may consist of immobilisation of the limb. However, the majority of authors consider this to be a professional error.

In some cases, where there is pain, non-steroidal anti-inflammatory drugs (NSAIDS) may be given, such as carprofen (4 mg/kg/day), ketoprofen (1 mg/kg/day), tepoxalin (10 mg/kg/day) or firocoxib (5 mg/kg/day). Chondroprotective agents are also indicated, to modify the course of the disease and help to re-establish joint function, improving mobility. These include symptomatic slow acting drugs for osteoarthritis (SYSADOA): hyaluronic acid, condroitin sulphate and glucosamine; and disease modifying osteoarthritis drug (DMOAD): hyaluronic acid and condroitin sulphate. These substances stimulate the condrocytes to increase extracellular matrix synthesis and block the wearing action of catabolic enzymes, thus altering the course of the disease and restoring joint function.

Patients not meeting the above criteria should be treated surgically. The choice of technique will depend on each individual case.

The prognosis for normal joint function in animals with ED is reserved, as progressive osteoarthritic changes can still be expected after any form of treatment.

The following is a description of each separate process, highlighting the aetiology, diagnosis, treatment and prognosis for each.

01 Fragmented coronoid process (FCP)

FCP is a common pathology of the elbow in large breeds of dog. During clinical examination the possibility of concurrent OCD must be considered; clinically it is difficult to differentiate between the two conditions and they often occur simultaneously. Suggested etiologies are the presence of osteochondrosis, local overloading or a general weakening of the cartilage and bone combined with mechanical overload.

The medial coronoid process is susceptible to fragmentation given that it is entirely formed by cartilage, and that its ossification is completed later than the other joint surfaces of the elbow. The chondrocytes located in the deepest layers do not survive as a result of the short supply of essential nutrients for cells to survive, as these substances cannot penetrate the thickened cartilage. This translates into fissures and splintering of the hyaline cartilage, affecting the subchondral bone. This is the most common cause of osteoarthritis of the elbow in the Rottweiler (74.9 %).

X-ray diagnosis of FCP is complex, given the difficulty in viewing the coronoid process on conventional X-ray images. For this reason, from a diagnosis point of view it is important to assess the secondary osteoarticular changes associated with the coronoid pathology.

The recommended positions for obtaining clear X-ray images allowing an early diagnosis of the coronoid process are caudomedial and craniolateral, at an oblique angle of 15°. The moderate overlap of the proximal epiphyses of the radius and ulna ensure an acceptable view of the medial coronoid apophysis on X-ray.

The possibility of visualising the joint using computerised axial tomography (CAT) enables an earlier and more precise diagnosis of the condition.

The treatment of choice for animals with FCP consists of removal of the coronoid process, approaching from the behind the round pronator or more caudally from behind the flexor carpi radialis muscle and in front of the superficial digital flexor muscle; or more recently using arthroscopic surgery.

Medical and surgical treatment can be offered with an equal degree of efficacy in dogs presenting lameness attributed to FCP.

The surgical technique of exeresis is currently the most universally accepted method by all authors, notwithstanding emerging techniques such as SHO (sliding humeral osteotomy) proposed by Fitzpatrick, with promising results.

Both FCP and OCD have a reserved prognosis, as claudication frequently persists and in the majority of cases the condition develops into a degenerative disease. Surgical treatment of FCP performed early in the life of the animal does not improve prognosis, however it does have an advantage over surgery performed on a joint in the advanced stage of the condition. Treatment with medication is also necessary, using NSAIDS and chondroprotectors.

02 Osteochondrosis dissecans (OCD)

The term **osteochondrosis dissecans** refers to the alteration of the endochondral ossification process resulting in the separation of a portion of the joint cartilage, previously known as osteochondritis dissecans.

OCD starts with the abnormal development of the joint cartilage, and an area of hypertrophy appears, leading to a longitudinal increase in the growth plate and a thickening of the cartilage itself. The cartilage becomes more sensitive to friction, after a time resulting in an area of variable size in which the subchondral bone comes away or dries out, forming a flap that either remains partially connected or completely breaks away from the surface of the bone, floating freely in the articular space.

The diagnosis of OCD presents difficulties similar to those for FCP; in this case the definitive X-ray observation is the appearance of an area of subchondral osteolysis in the medial part of the humeral condyle. Occasionally a detachment and typical chronic osteoarthritic changes can be seen.

As regards the treatment of OCD in the elbow joint, as is the case with this condition in other joints, it can be corrected by the surgical removal of the cartilaginous flap and by drilling holes (foraging) in the crater of the damaged area, thus encouraging the growth of fibrous cartilage tissue, which is less resistant than hyaline. Hyaline tissue does not regenerate.

As already mentioned above, the prognosis is reserved given the progress of the degenerative condition, the presence of persistent claudication and the need to administer adjuvant medication.

03 Ununited anconeal process (UAP)

The aetiology of **UAP** is not at all clear. A number of different factors have been considered, such as hereditary growth anomalies, or metabolic and nutritional alterations and growth hormone alterations. However, it has been established that it results from a failure of the fourth nucleus of ossification to bind with the metaphysis. Trauma to the joint are also considered to be a causal factor.

The diagnosis of UAP presents the least number of complications. It can be swiftly recognised by taking a mediolateral X-ray of the elbow joint in flexion, separating the image of the anconeal process from that of the humeral epicondyle, which otherwise would overlap. X-ray diagnosis is based on the presence of a radiotransparent line separating the anconeal process from the proximal ulnar epiphysis. Although this pathology is generally clear enough not to present complications in diagnosis, on occasions the line of separation may be very faint. This does not necessarily indicated that fusion is underway, but denotes the presence of strong bands of connective tissue that hold the anconeal process in position. This condition can only be diagnosed after the age of 5 months, at which time the synostosis of the two structures takes place.

Elbow joints presenting UAP should be examined to identify any concurrent pathologies that may affect recovery. The condition commonly affects the German Shepherd and is the easiest to diagnose of all the pathologies making up ED.

UAP has been treated using fixation, removal or proximal ulnar osteotomy.

04 Joint incongruity (JI)

The humeroradioulnar joint loses its anatomical harmony as a result of different alterations in the growth of the bones that comprise it, for example, shortening of the radius, the ulna or both, a poor fit between the rim of the trochlear notch and the trochlear of the humerus, or premature closure of growth lines resulting from direct trauma to the area. These alterations lead to angular deformities (Figs. 8, 9 and 10).

This causes abnormal loads on different areas of the joint surfaces and undue friction on the cartilage, resulting in degenerative joint disease. Joint incongruity of the elbow joint contributes to the pathogenesis of UAP and FCP, and is bilateral in 50 % of affected animals. Where both limbs are compromised, claudication may be erratic, initially indiscernible or evident only after exercise. Some dog owners report rigidity when walking, in particular in the mornings after intense physical activity. However, some dogs show more intense symptoms after periods of inactivity. While walking, internal rotation of the elbow and carpal supination are observed during extension or moving forward.

The clinical examination reveals pain on extreme flexion and extension, and at times crepitation and clear effusion between the lateral epicondyle and the anconeal process. In longer established cases, examination shows moderate muscular atrophy of the forelimb.

It is suggested that the diagnosis of JI is based on the observation of the following alterations under X-ray, reflected in Table 2.

Table 2. X-ray alterations in joint incongruity.

- Abnormal shape of trochlear notch.
- Enlarged, irregular or assymetrical articular spaces.
- Alteration of congruity between the articular surface of the notch and that of the radius (radioulnar step).
- Osteophytes on the dorsal surface of anconeal process.
- Irregular edge of the coronoid process.

Treatment of JI depends on the underlying causal pathology. If there is malformation of the trochlear notch, only symptomatic treatment can be given, together with treatment for subsequent resulting FCP and UAP. JI caused by asynchronous radioulnar growth is treated with transverse or oblique ulnar osteotomy/ostectomy via a caudal approach. A Steinmann pin is inserted from the olecranon across the line of osteotomy into the distal portion of the ulna, thus securing the correct alignment of the bone shaft.

The prognosis for JI depends on the severity of the changes to the joint surfaces of the bones of the joint, the possibility of surgical correction and the time at which treatment is given. In some cases Fitzpatrick's SHO (Sliding Humeral Osteotomy) may be effective in relieving the excess load on the joint. In any event, the prognosis varies from reserved to unfavourable, and adjuvant medical treatment is habitually required.

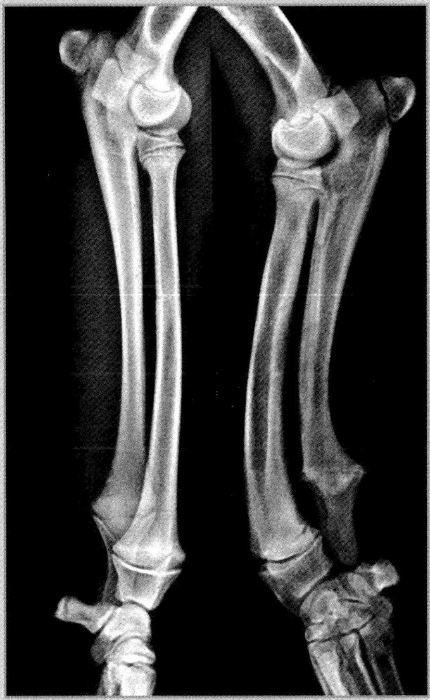

Figure 8. Joint incongruity due to trapped distal ulna growth cartilage.

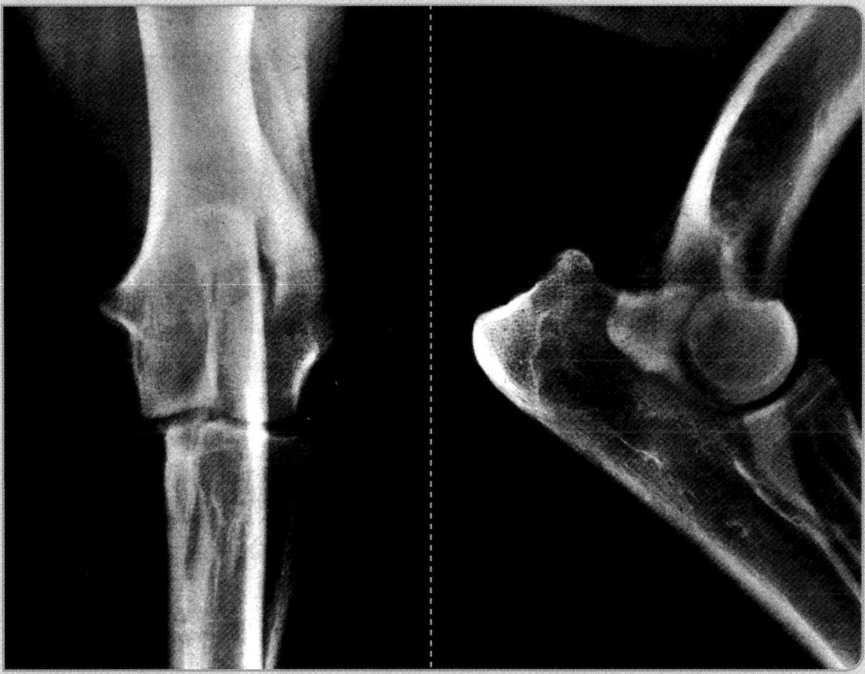

Figure 9. Incomplete ossification of the humeral condyle. Difficult to diagnose by X-ray.

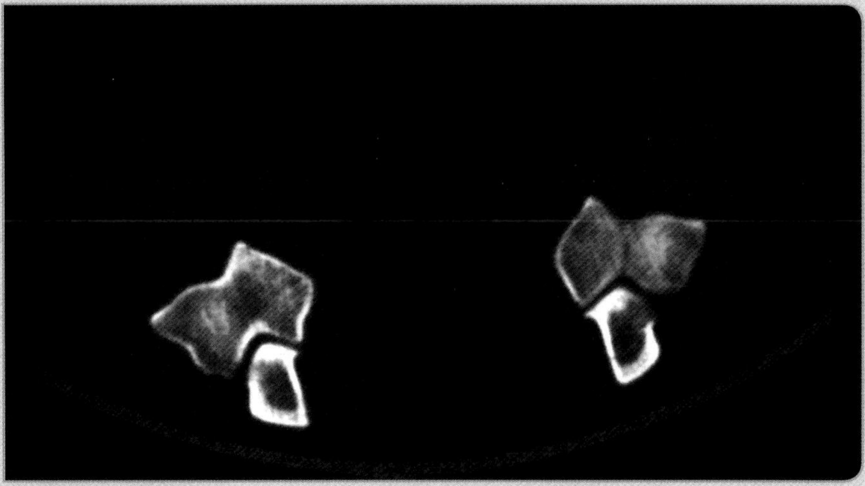

Figure 10. Incomplete ossification of the humeral condyle in a 7 year old German Shorthaired Pointer. CAT image.

Diagnostic imaging techniques

The following are pairs of images comparing transparent plastinated sections of real structures compared with images obtained using CAT and MRI.

Transparent plastinated sections + CAT

SAGITTAL SECTION OF THE ELBOW JOINT IN SEMI-FLEXION

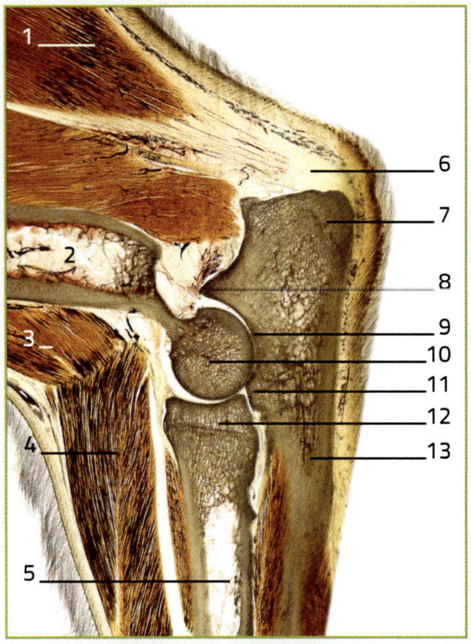

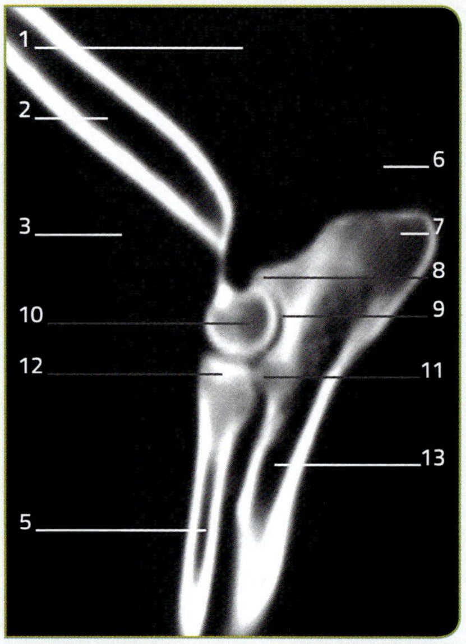

1	Triceps brachii muscle
2	Shaft of humerus
3	Biceps brachii muscle
4	Extensor carpi radialis muscle
5	Shaft of radius
6	Tendon of insertion of triceps brachii muscle
7	Olecranon tuberosity
8	Anconeal apophysis
9	Trochlear notch
10	Condyle of the humerus, capitulum
11	Lateral coronoid apophysis
12	Head of radius
13	Ulna

OBLIQUE TRANSVERSAL SECTION OF THE ELBOW JOINT

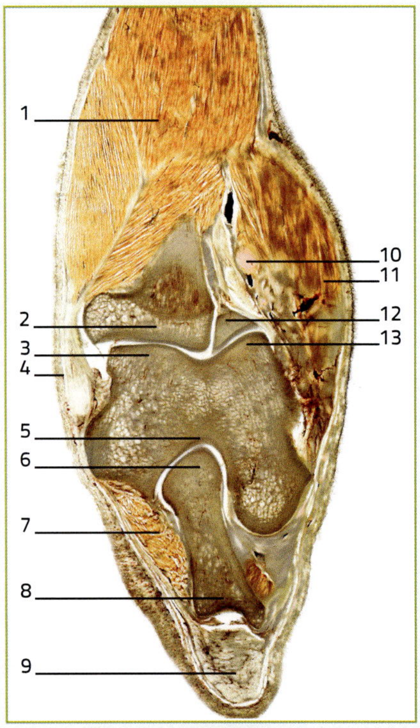

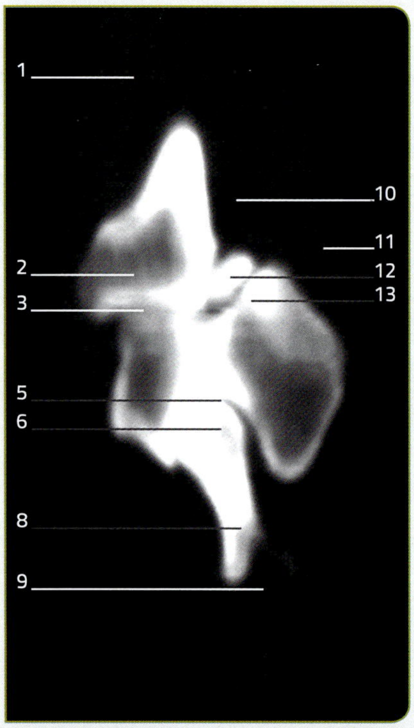

1	Extensor carpi radialis muscle
2	Head of radius
3	Condyle of the humerus, capitulum
4	Lateral collateral lig.
5	Olecranon fossa
6	Anconeal apophysis
7	Anconeal muscle
8	Olecranon tuberosity
9	Tendon of insertion of triceps brachii muscle
10	Brachial artery
11	Pronator teres muscle
12	Medial coronoid apophysis
13	Condyle of the humerus, trochlea

Transparent plastinated sections + MRI

SAGITTAL SECTION OF THE ELBOW JOINT IN SEMI-FLEXION

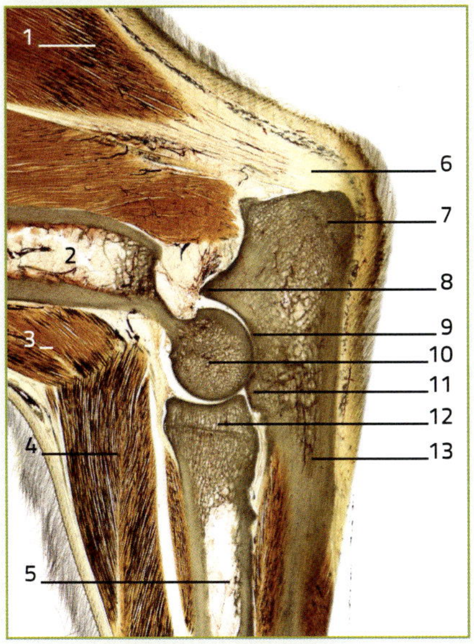

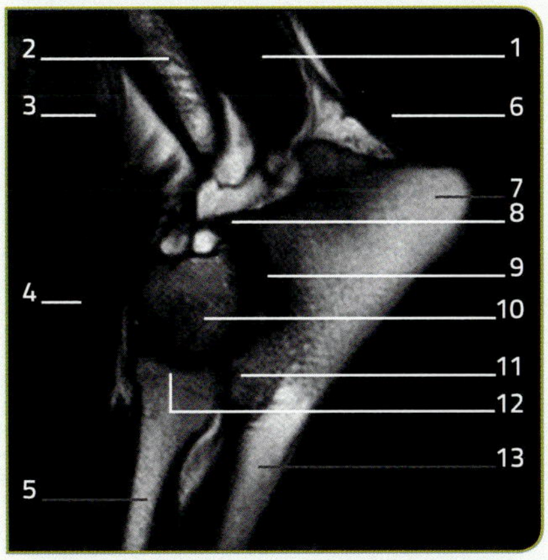

1	Triceps brachii muscle
2	Shaft of humerus
3	Biceps brachii muscle
4	Extensor carpi radialis muscle
5	Shaft of radius
6	Tendon of insertion of triceps brachii muscle
7	Olecranon tuberosity
8	Anconeal apophysis
9	Trochlear notch
10	Condyle of the humerus, capitulum
11	Lateral coronoid apophysis
12	Head of radius
13	Ulna

OBLIQUE TRANSVERSAL SECTION OF THE ELBOW JOINT

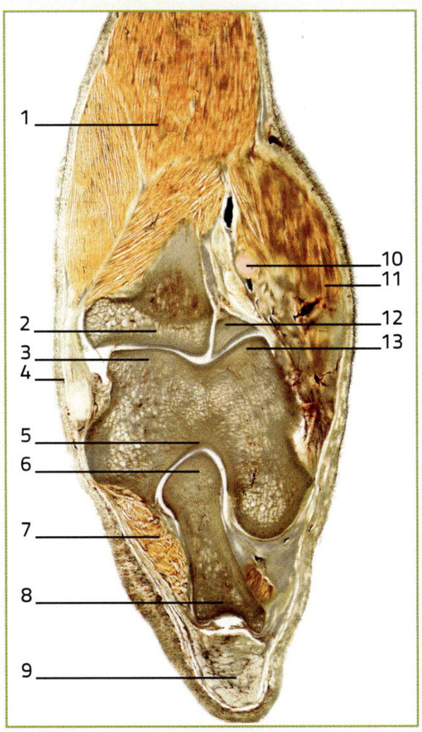

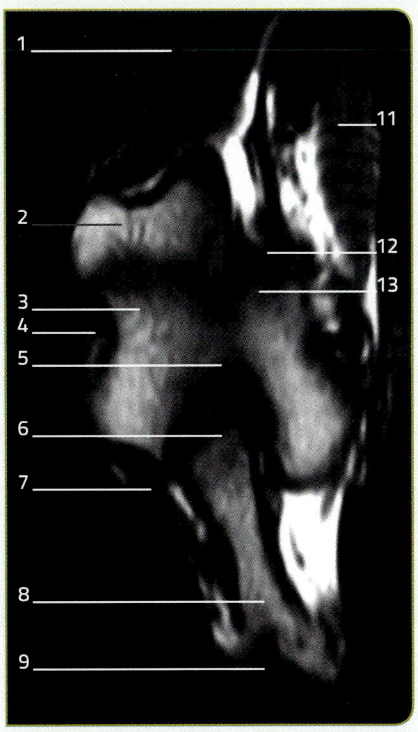

1	Extensor carpi radialis muscle
2	Head of radius
3	Condyle of the humerus, capitulum
4	Lateral collateral lig.
5	Olecranon fossa
6	Anconeal apophysis
7	Anconeal muscle
8	Olecranon tuberosity
9	Tendon of insertion of triceps brachii muscle
10	Brachial artery
11	Pronator teres muscle
12	Medial coronoid apophysis
13	Condyle of the humerus, trochlea

SURGICAL APPROACHES

Approach to the lateral side of the humeral condyle and epicondyle

1 The skin incision extends from the distal third of the humerus to the proximal third of the forearm, passing over the lateral humeral epicondyle. After sectioning the fascia of the forelimb, the line separating the extensor carpi radialis and common digital extensor muscles is identified to obtain deeper access into this space. The course of the radial nerve must be respected.

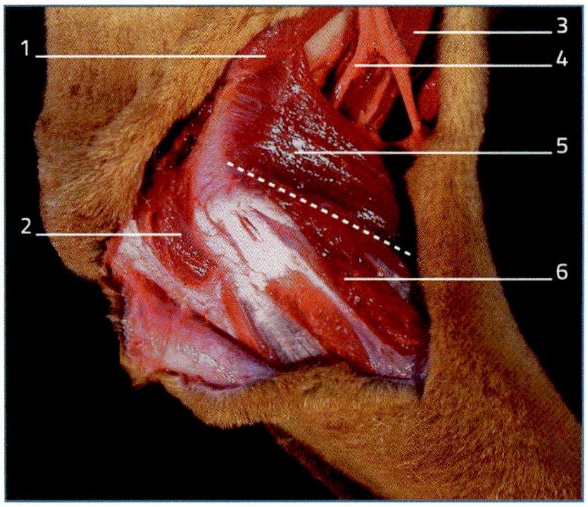

1 Triceps brachii muscle, lateral head
2 Anconeal muscle
3 Brachial muscle
4 Radial nerve
5 Extensor carpi radialis muscle
6 Common digital extensor muscle

2 The laterocranial surface of the joint and the supinator muscle are exposed by displacing the extensor carpi radialis muscle cranially and the common digital extensor muscle caudally. Forced supination of the forearm helps exposure of the joint.

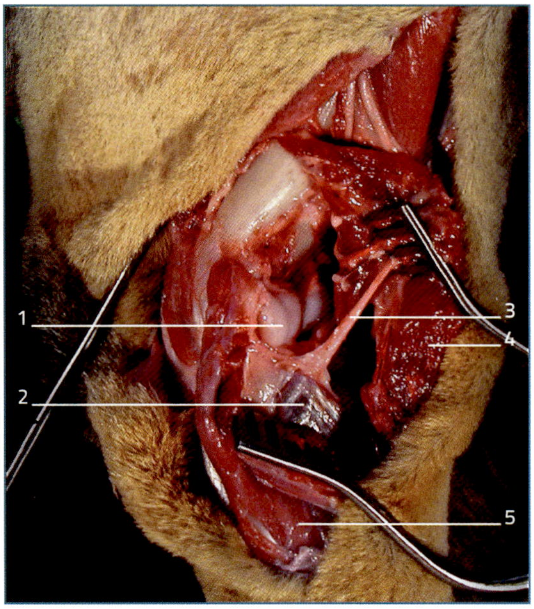

1 Condyle of the humerus
2 Supinator muscle
3 Radial nerve
4 Extensor carpi radialis muscle
5 Common digital extensor muscle

Approach to the supracondylar region of the humerus and the caudal humeroulnar portion of the elbow joint

1 A curved incision is made over the olecranon fossa, between the lateral humeral epicondyle and the olecranon tuberosity.

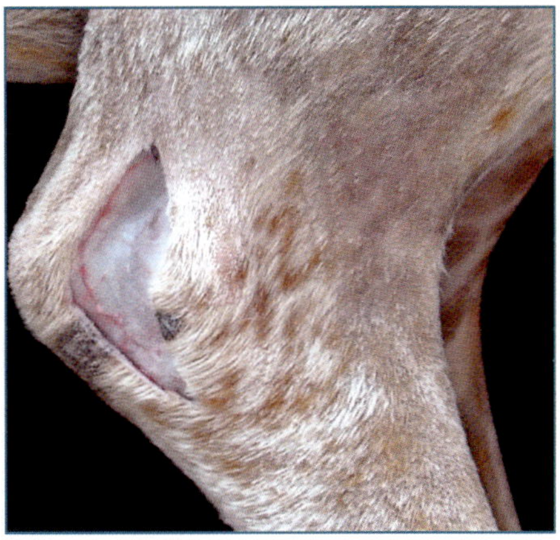

2 After sectioning the fascia of the elbow, the tendon of insertion of the triceps brachii muscle and the edges of the anconeal muscle are located. The latter must be detached from its caudal attachment to the ulna.

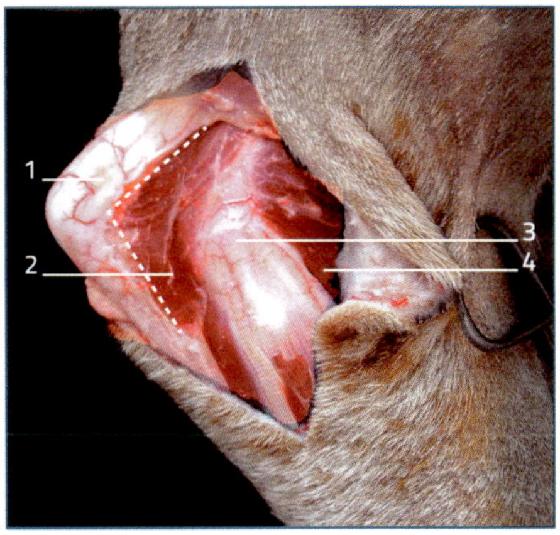

1 Triceps brachii muscle tendon
2 Anconeal muscle
3 Lateral epicondyle of the humerus
4 Extensor carpi radialis muscle

3 Detachment of the anconeal muscle allows the caudal part of the joint to be located. Flexion of the joint and medial displacement of the triceps brachii tendon provides a better view of the anconeal apophysis and the olecranon fossa.

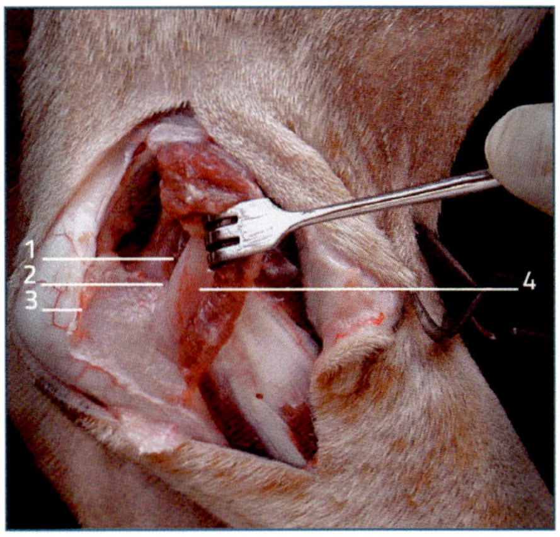

1 Olecranon fossa
2 Anconeal apophysis
3 Olecranon tuberosity
4 Lateral epicondyle of the humerus

Approach to the humeroulnar portion of the elbow joint via osteotomy of the olecranon

1 The skin incision is made between the supracondylar region of the humerus and the caudal humeroulnar portion of the elbow joint. The edges of the anconeal muscle are then located in order to detach it from the ulna.

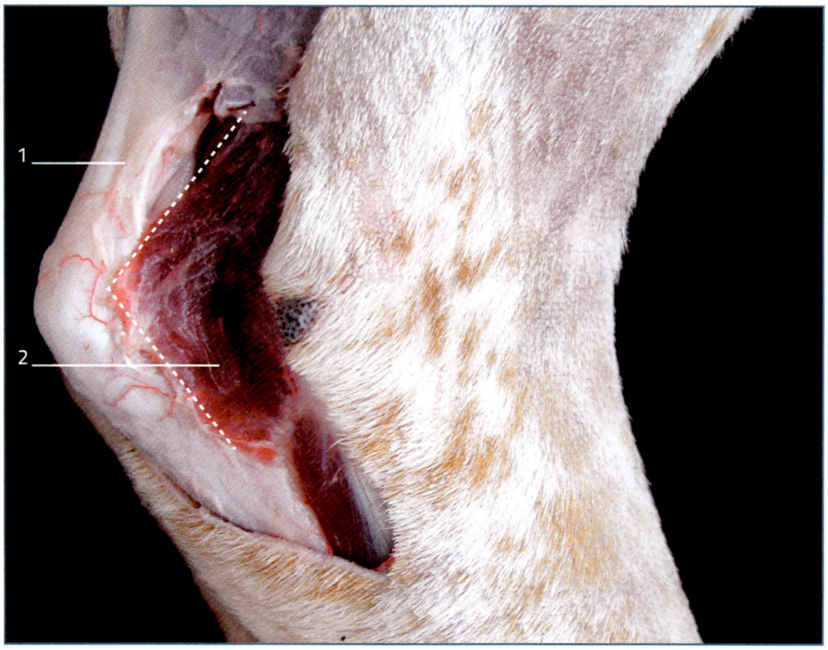

1 Triceps brachii muscle tendon
2 Anconeal muscle

2 Cranial displacement of the anconeal muscle allows location of the triceps brachii muscle and the surface of the olecranon tuberosity, which is sectioned at an angle of 45° during the osteotomy. The course of the ulnar nerve must be respected.

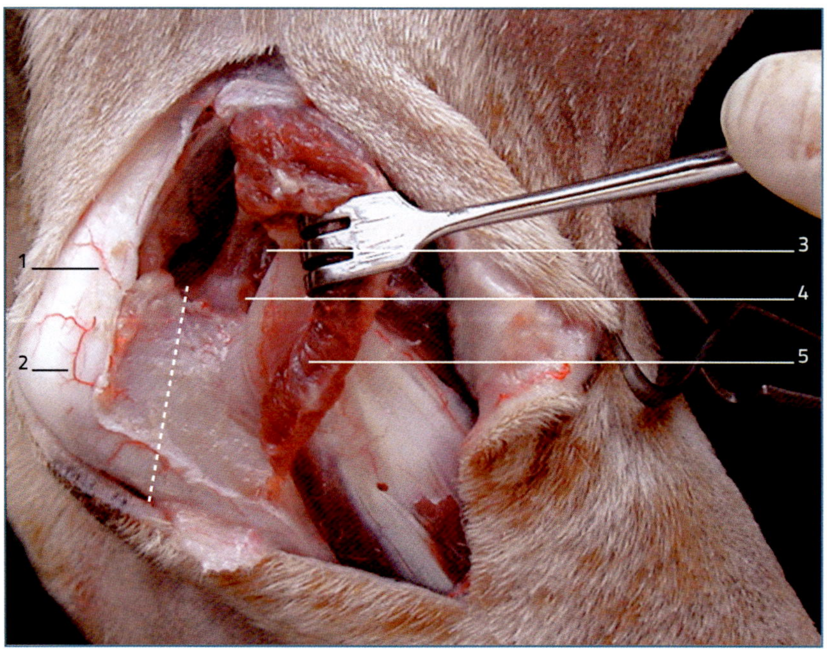

1 Triceps brachii muscle tendon
2 Olecranon tuberosity
3 Olecranon fossa
4 Anconeal apophysis
5 Anconeal muscle

3 After osteotomy of the olecranon tuberosity, a caudal approach is taken to the joint, separating the olecranon tuberosity and the triceps brachii tendon.

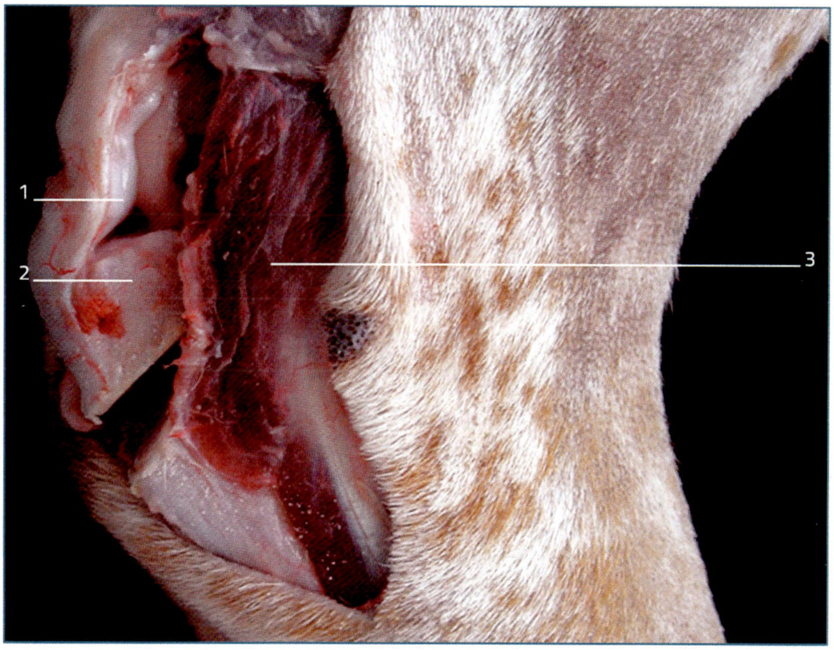

1 Triceps brachii muscle tendon
2 Olecranon tuberosity
3 Anconeal muscle

4 The joint problems are exposed caudally by displacing the olecranon and the triceps brachii muscle tendon towards the proximal area. The anconeal apophysis and the olecranon fossa are clearly identifiable upon forcing flexion of the joint.

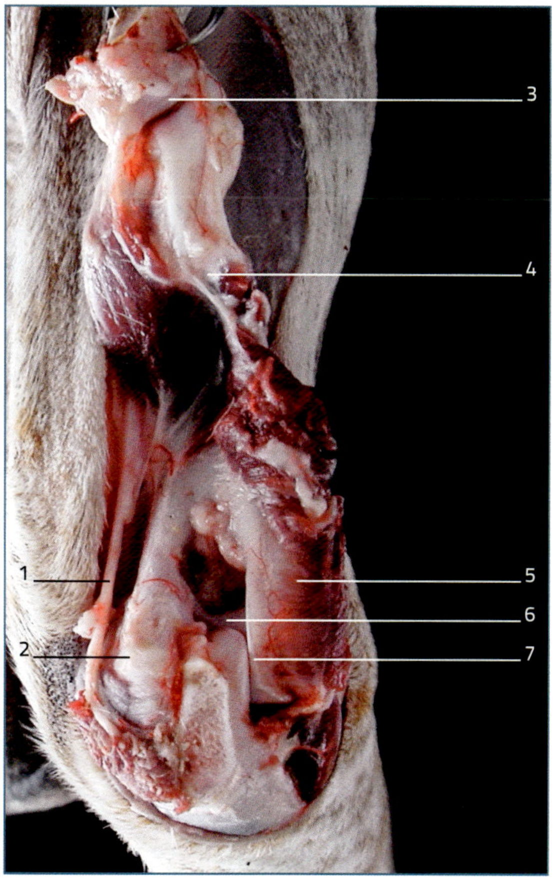

1 Ulnar nerve
2 Medial epicondyle
3 Olecranon tuberosity
4 Triceps brachii tendon and muscle
5 Anconeal muscle
6 Anconeal apophysis
7 Lateral epicondyle

Approach to the medial surface of the humeral condyle and medial coronoid apophysis of the ulna via intermuscular incision

1 The skin incision extends in a curve from the distal third of the humerus to the proximal third of the forearm, passing over the medial epicondyle of the humerus.

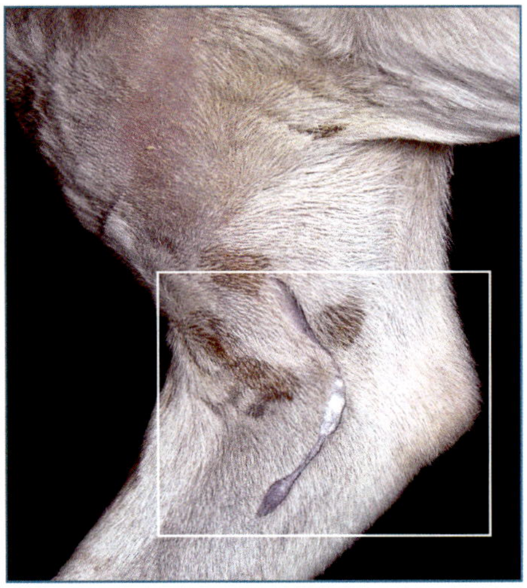

2 After drawing back the skin the fascia of the forearm and the course of the ulnar nerve can be located. The fascia must be sectioned to access flexor muscles of the forearm.

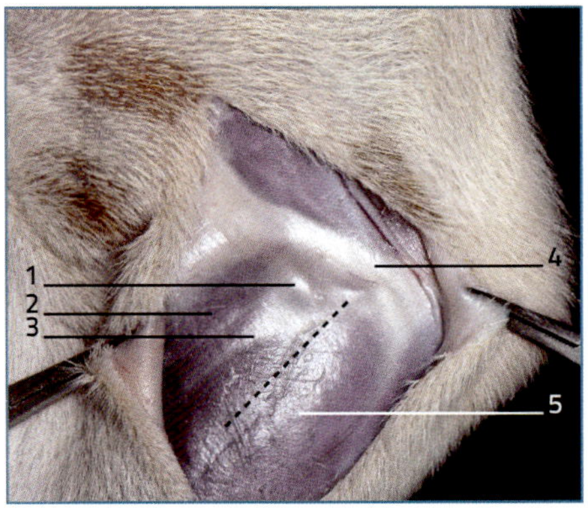

1 Medial epicondyle of the humerus
2 Pronator teres muscle
3 Fascia of the forearm
4 Ulnar nerve
5 Superficial digital flexor muscle

3 After sectioning the fascia of the forearm the line of separation between the flexor carpi radialis and superficial digital flexor muscles is located. An incision along this intramuscular line allows a medial approach to the joint.

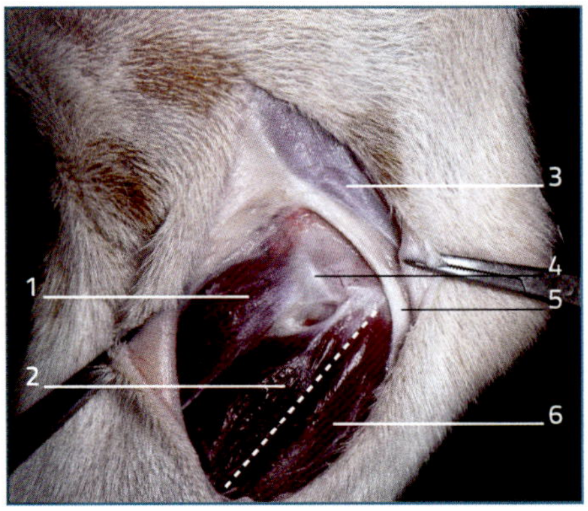

1 Pronator teres muscle
2 Flexor carpi radialis muscle
3 Triceps brachii muscle
4 Medial epicondyle of the humerus
5 Ulnar nerve
6 Superficial digital flexor muscle

4 Cranial displacement of the flexor carpi radialis muscle and caudal displacement of the superficial digital flexor muscle exposes the joint.

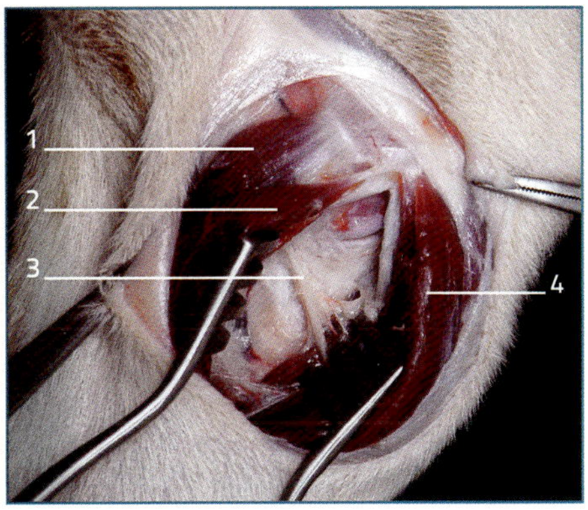

1 Pronator teres muscle
2 Flexor carpi radialis muscle
3 Muscular branches of the median nerve
4 Superficial digital flexor muscle

5 The articular edges are located by partially sectioning the articular capsule. The collateral medial ligament is also seen in the most cranial area of the approach. In the distal area, the tendon of insertion of the biceps brachii and brachial muscles can be seen.

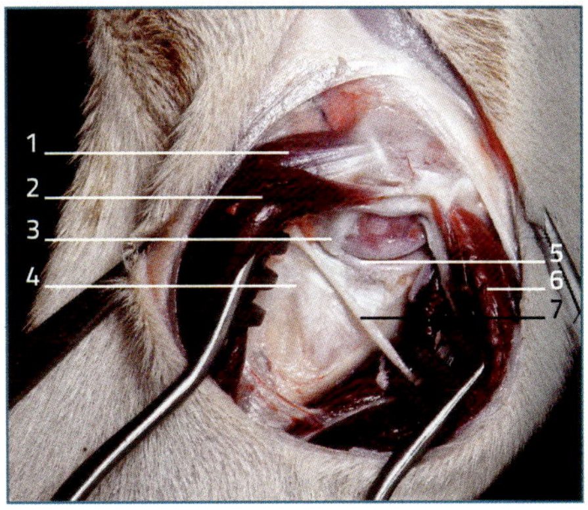

1 Pronator teres muscle
2 Flexor carpi radialis muscle
3 Medial collateral ligament
4 Tendon of the biceps brachii and brachial muscles
5 Medial coronoid apophysis
6 Superficial digital flexor muscle
7 Muscular branches of the median nerve

6 Enlargement of the area after forcing pronation or internal rotation of the forearm with abduction. This makes it possible to expose the articular surface of the medial coronoid process.

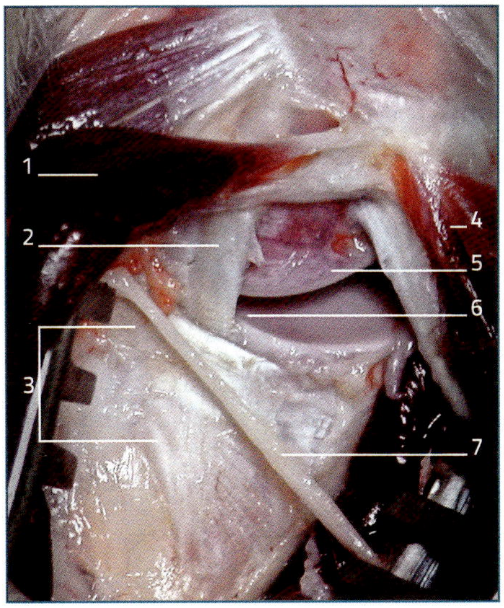

1 Flexor carpi radialis muscle
2 Medial collateral ligament
3 Tendon of the biceps brachii and brachial muscles
4 Superficial digital flexor muscle
5 Humeral condyle trochlea
6 Medial coronoid apophysis
7 Muscular branches of the median nerve

The images included for surgical approaches are adapted from: Latorre, R., Gil, F., Climent, S., López, O., Henry, R., Ayala, M., Ramírez, G., Martínez, F., Vázquez, J.M. *Color Atlas of Surgical Approaches to the Bones and Joints of the Dog and Cat*. Intermédica S.A., 2009; pp. 0-266. ISBN 978-950-555-353-2.

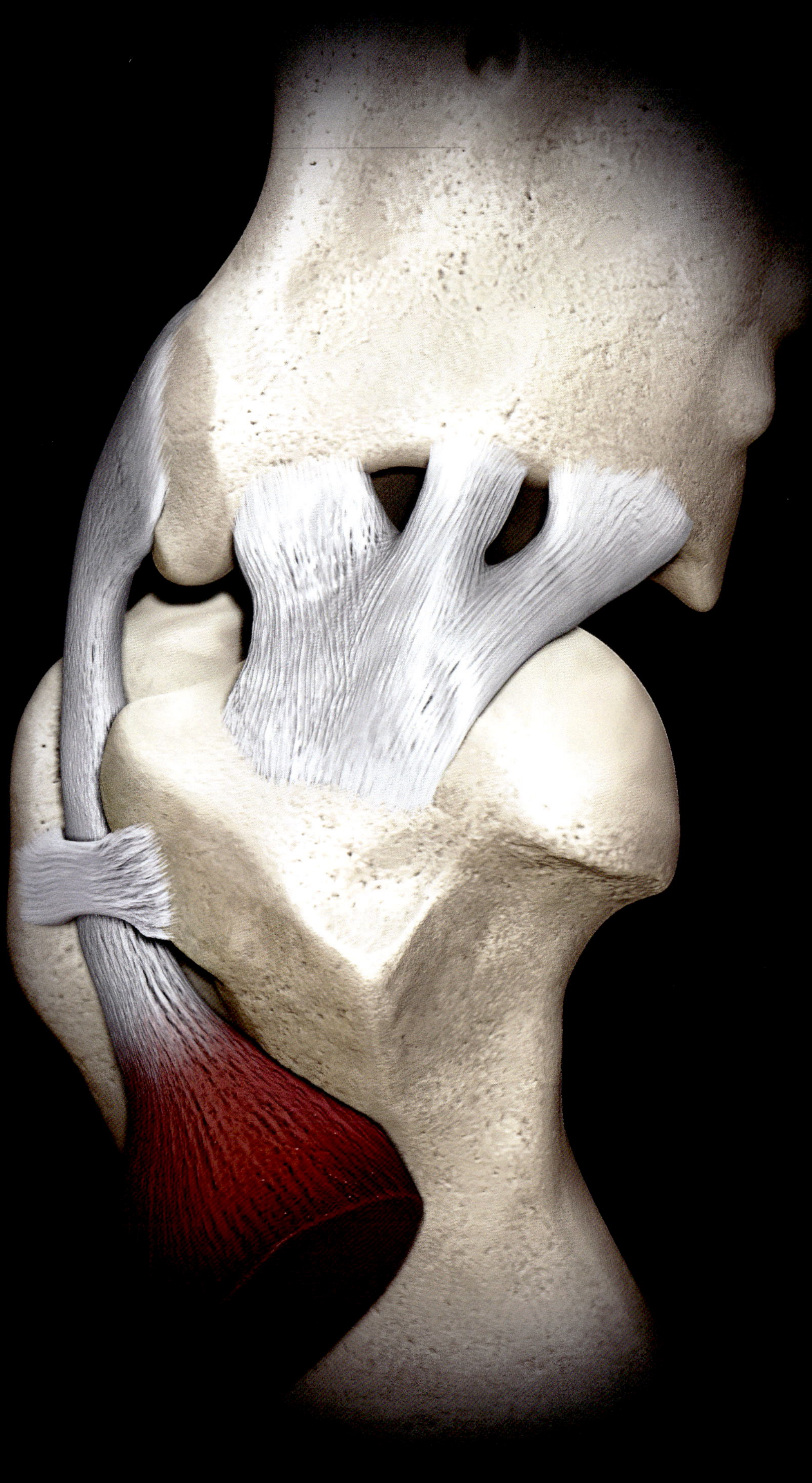

SHOULDER JOINT

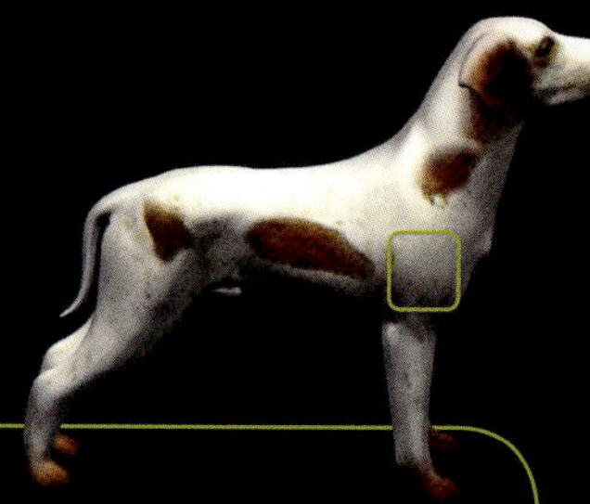

Shoulder joint

LATERAL VIEW

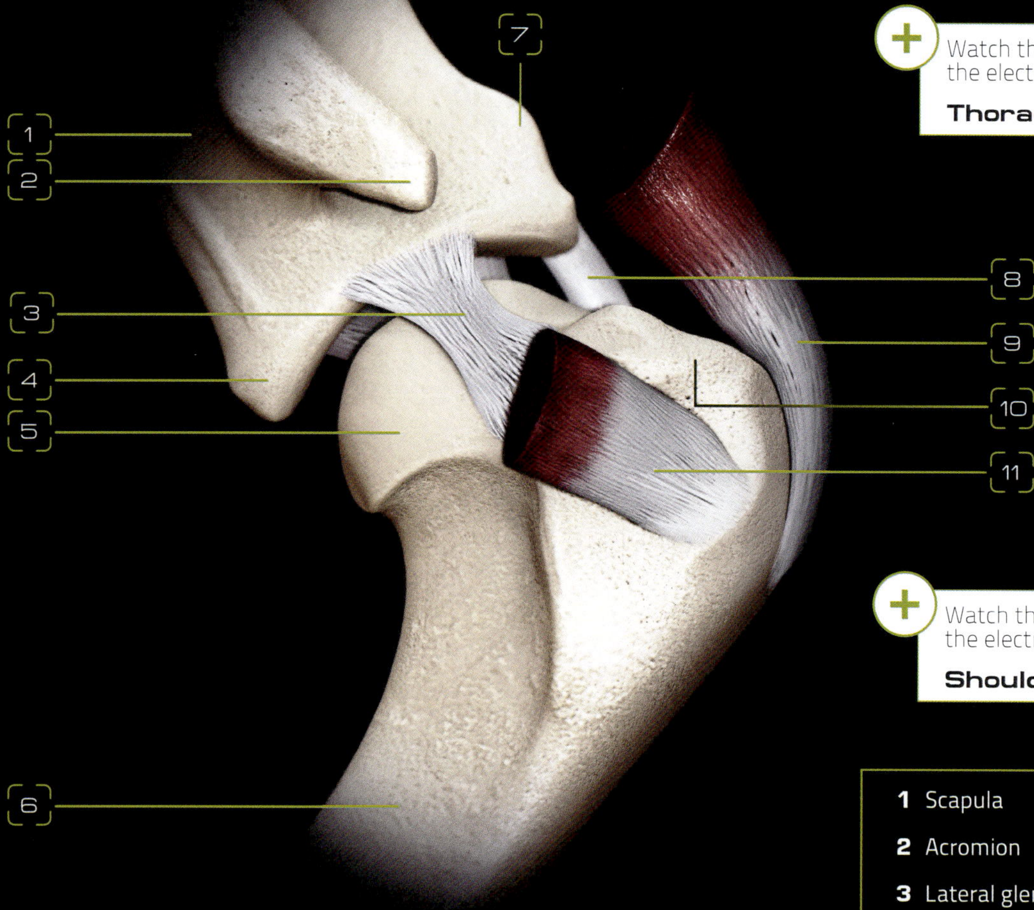

+ Watch this video on the electronic version
Thoracic limb

+ Watch this video on the electronic version
Shoulder joint

LATERAL VIEW WITH EXTERNAL HUMERAL ROTATION

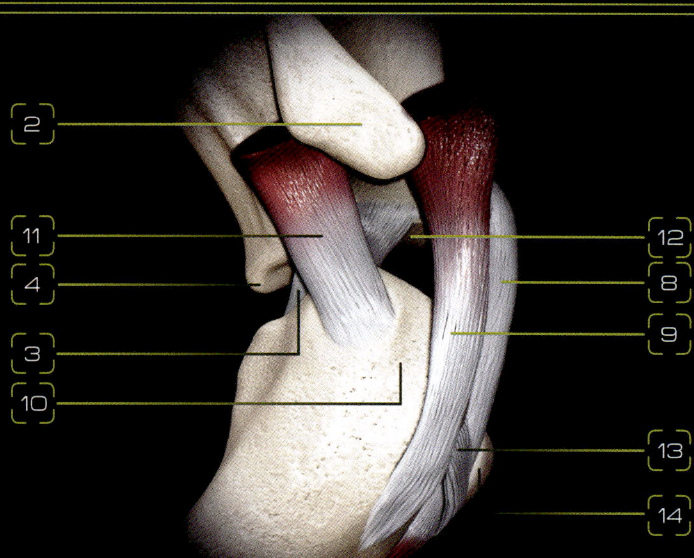

1 Scapula
2 Acromion
3 Lateral glenohumeral lig.
4 Infraglenoid tubercle
5 Head of humerus
6 Humerus
7 Supraglenoid tubercle
8 Tendon of the biceps brachii muscle
9 Tendon of the supraspinatus muscle
10 Greater tubercle of the humerus
11 Tendon of the infraspinatus muscle
12 Glenoid cavity
13 Transverse lig. of the shoulder joint
14 Lesser tubercle of the humerus

MEDIAL VIEW

1 Subscapular fossa
2 Supraglenoid tubercle
3 Tendon of the biceps brachii muscle
4 Tendon of the supraspinatus muscle
5 Greater tubercle of the humerus
6 Transverse lig. of the shoulder joint
7 Medial glenohumeral lig.
8 Infraglenoid tubercle
9 Head of humerus
10 Lesser tubercle of the humerus

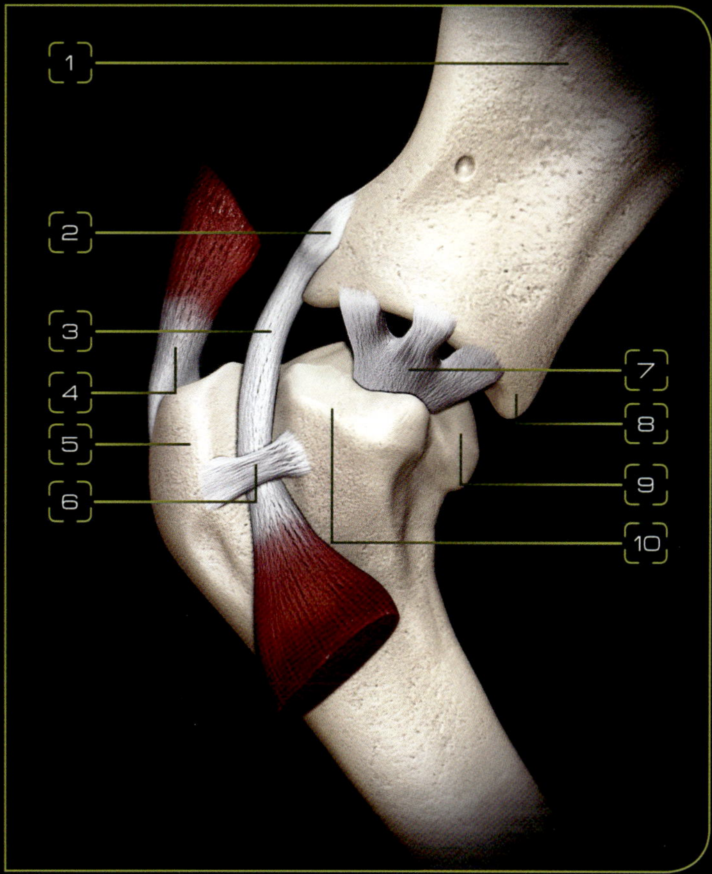

MEDIAL VIEW WITH EXTERNAL HUMERAL ROTATION

1 Supraglenoid tubercle
2 Coracoid apophysis
3 Tendon of the biceps brachii muscle
4 Lesser tubercle of the humerus
5 Transverse lig. of the shoulder joint
6 Infraglenoid tubercle
7 Medial glenohumeral lig.
8 Head of humerus

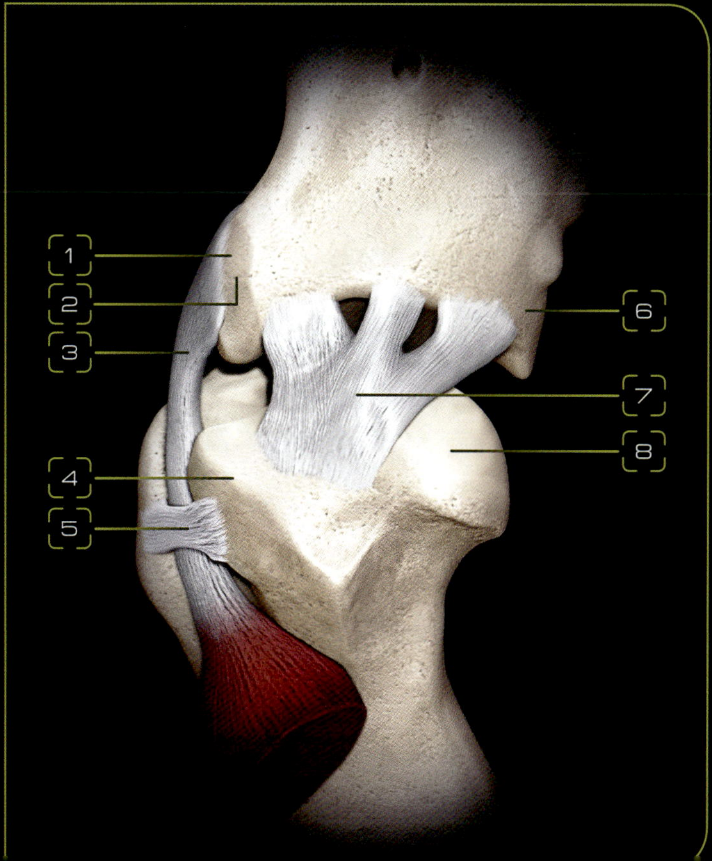

Orthopaedic conditions of the shoulder

The most common orthopaedic conditions of the shoulder joint are:

01 Luxations

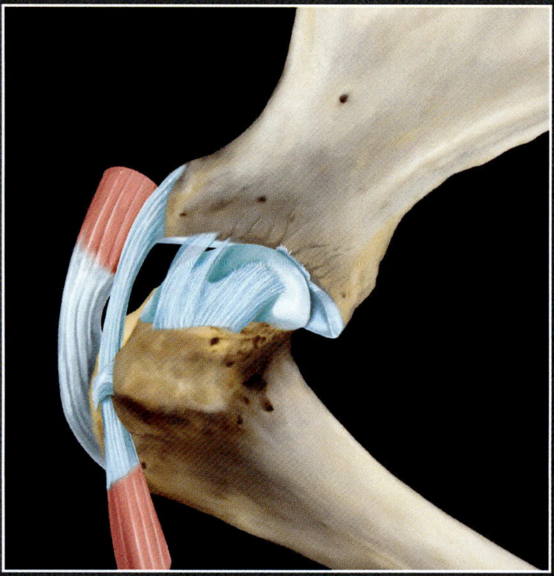

02 Osteochondrosis dissecans (OCD) of the humeral head

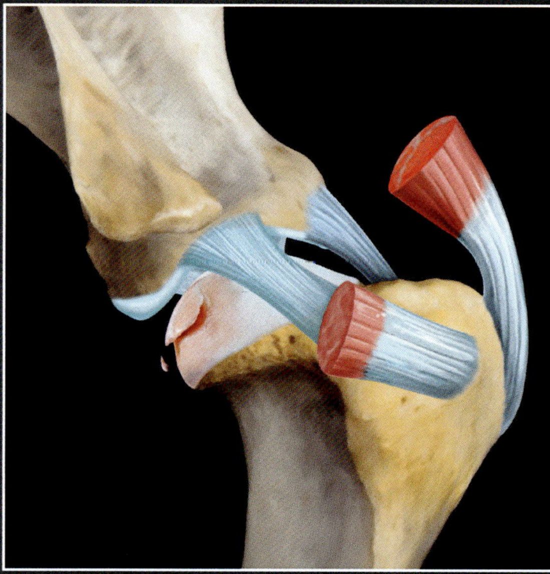

03 Calcification of the supraspinatus tendon

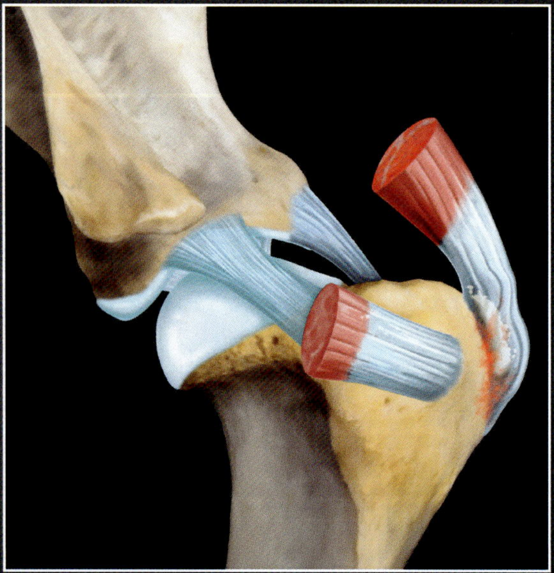

04 Tenosynovitis of biceps brachii muscle tendon

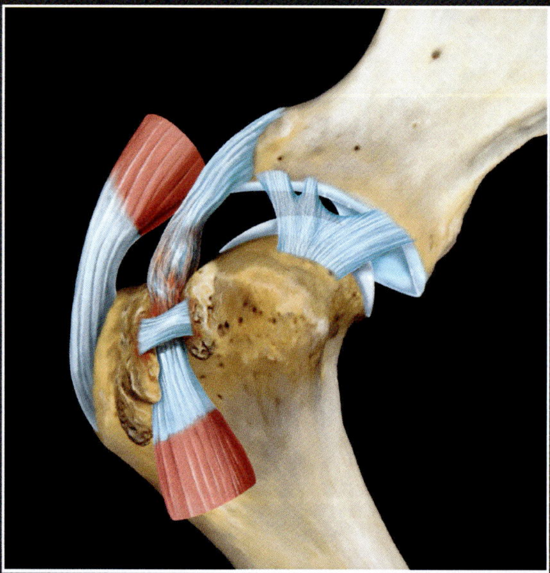

01

Luxations

Dorsal luxation of the scapula

Ruptures of the insertions of the serratis ventralis, trapezius and rhomboids muscles on the dorsal border of the scapula result in dorsal displacement when weight is placed on the limb. Scapular mobility is easily diagnosed.

Treatment consists of pinning the scapula to a rib with a cerclage and stitching of the ruptured muscles. The muscles can also be reinserted at the scapular via holes drilled close to the cranial angle.

Postoperatively the scapula is immobilised for two weeks using a Velpeau sling.

Luxations of the shoulder joint

The Miniature Poodle and the Shetland Sheepdog are particularly prone to suffering medial luxations without any prior trauma. The large majority (75 %) of luxations are medial, and the remainder lateral. Cranial and caudal luxations are only seen in exceptional cases. The most important stabilising ligaments are the glenohumeral ligaments and the joint capsule.

A stress X-ray is indicated as an objective method for diagnosing instability in this joint. If the glenoid cavity has been severely worn down by chronic luxation or dysplasia of the glenoid cavity or head of the humerus, successful reduction is less likely. Congenital luxations discovered at a late stage generally cannot be reduced.

Luxations can be congenital or traumatic, and are classified in terms of the direction of the dislocation; medial, lateral, cranial and caudal (Figs. 1, 2 and 3).

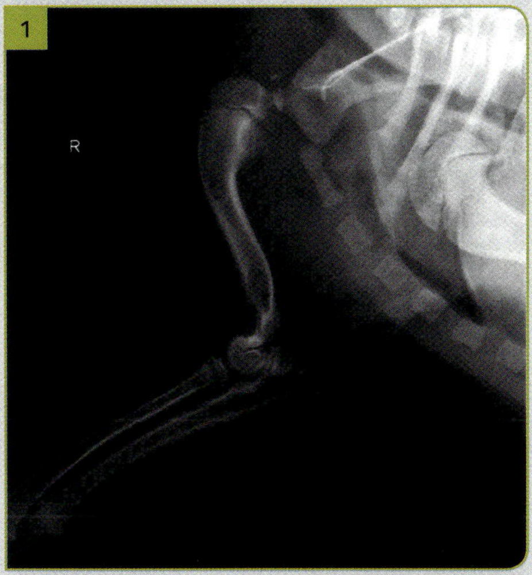

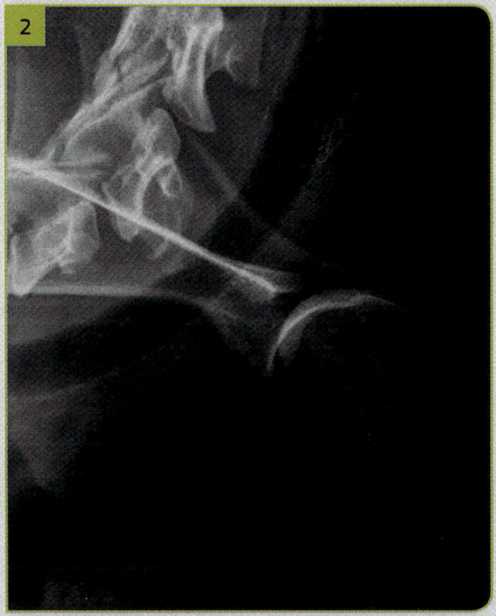

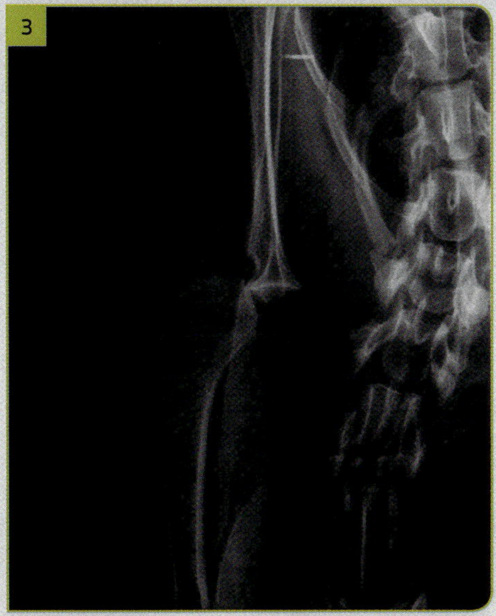

Figure 1. X-ray image of a cranial luxation of the shoulder.
Figure 2. X-ray image of a medial luxation of the shoulder.
Figure 3. X-ray image of a lateral luxation of the shoulder.

Medial luxation

If the glenoid cavity is deformed it makes no sense to attempt surgical stabilisation. In this case, excision arthroplasty or arthrodesis are more effective. If the joint surfaces are healthy and the luxation is recent, the joint can be stabilised by suturing the joint capsule and the subscapularis muscle tendon. If the tissues are damaged tenodesis of the biceps tendon is performed (Figs. 4, 5 and 6). This requires sectioning of the transverse humeral ligament. The tendon is then removed from the intertubercular groove after incising the joint capsule. A semi-lunate flap of bone from the lesser tuberosity is then prepared. This flap acts as a hinge on the periosteum with the cranial border. The tendon is moved caudally under the flap and fixed in this position using Kirschner wire.

Another tenodesis technique is to section the tendon and fix it to the humerus using a screw and a washer in a gentle depression of the periostium (Fig. 7).

The overlap of the joint capsule and the medial glenohumeral ligament is achieved using mattress sutures in a synthetic self-absorbing material. The deep pectoral muscle is sutured to the superficial pectoral muscle by moving the subscapularis muscle as far cranially as possible, and fixing it to the deep pectoral muscle. Finally the superficial pectoral muscle is placed along the cranial border of the humerus and sutured to the acromial head of the deltoid muscle. The effect of these changes in muscle position is to tighten and strengthen the medial support of the joint.

Postoperative care consists of a Velpeau sling worn for 14 days. Exercise should be limited for 4 weeks. After this time physiotherapy can commence, including swimming where possible.

Lateral luxation

Lateral luxations are seen most commonly in large breeds and are generally trauma induced. Conservative treatment can be successful in these cases. In the case of chronic luxations or where reduction is not possible, the biceps muscle tenodesis technique can be used. This is performed by osteotomy of the greater tuberosity of the humerus. The lateral lip of the glenoid cavity and the medial surface of the humeral head must always be examined carefully. If these structures are compromised, excision arthroplasty or arthrodesis may be more successful.

If the joint surfaces are in good condition and the luxation is recent, the joint can be stabilised with sutures through the joint capsule. If this option is not considered appropriate, biceps tendon tenodesis is indicated.

The technique for exposing this tendon is similar to that described for medial luxation, except that the tendon is moved towards the lateral area. The tendon moved laterally to the remaining crest of the greater tuberosity. The tendon is then held laterally while the humeral tubercle is pinned using Kirschner wires. The joint capsule is fixed using mattress or Lembert sutures. The superficial pectoral muscle is moved craniolaterally and joined to the deltoid and biceps muscle fascia.

Postoperative care for this procedure is the same as that described for medial luxation.

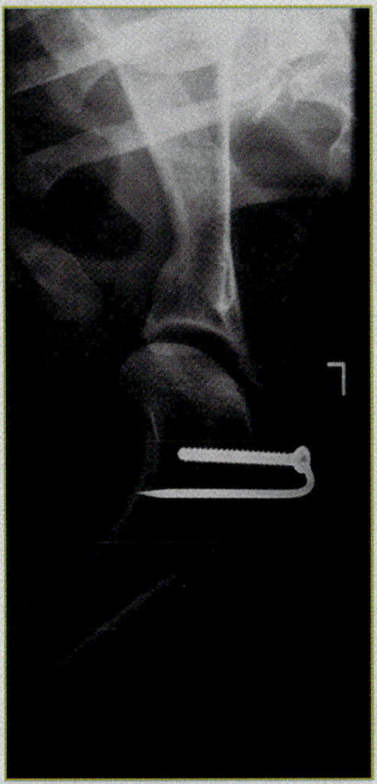

Figure 4. Surgical treatment involving repositioning of the biceps tendon.

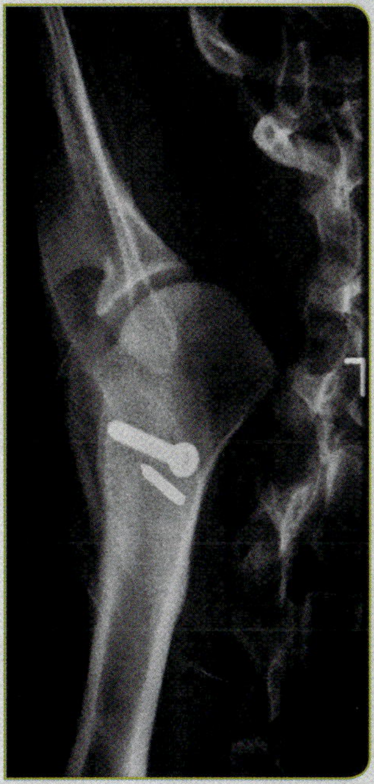

Figure 5. Craniocaudal view of surgical treatment involving repositioning of the biceps tendon.

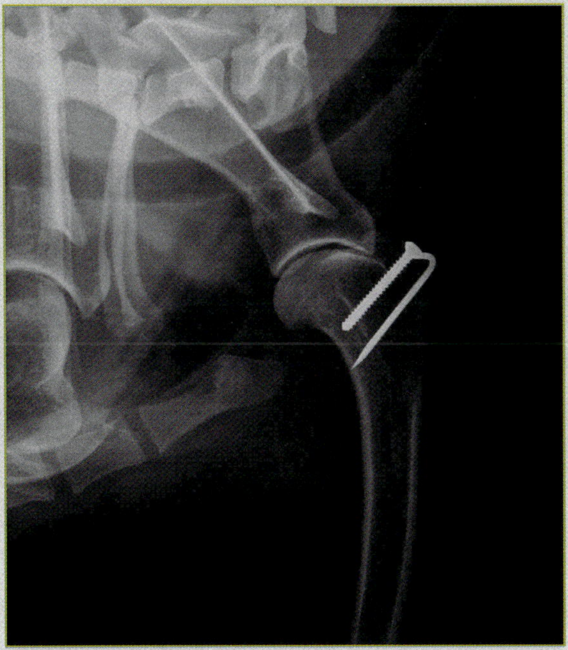

Figure 6. X-ray image after 8 weeks.

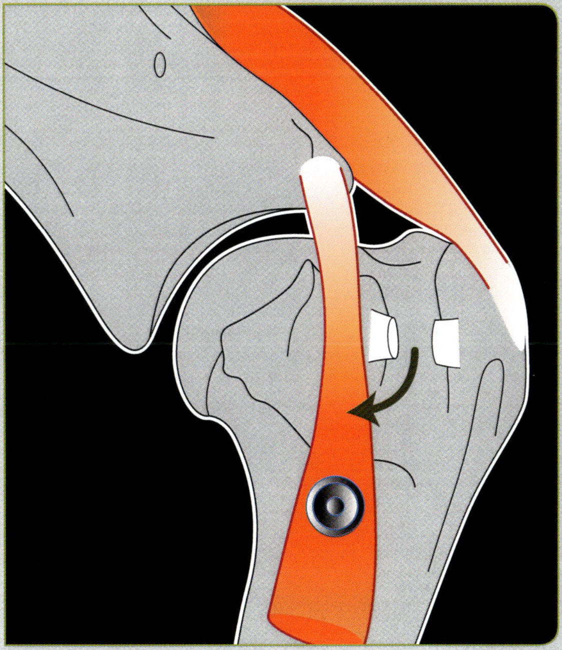

Figure 7. Diagram of the surgical technique of tenodesis of the biceps tendon.

02 Osteochondrosis dissecans (OCD) of the humeral head

Osteochondrosis is an alteration of cell differentiation on the metaphyseal growth plate and joint cartilage. Generally speaking, the cartilage in the lower layers does not mature into bone tissue in a uniform manner. This results in local areas of thickening in the cartilage, and synovial nutrition is lost (Figs. 8 and 9). If a flap forms in the joint cartilage with joint inflammation, this is known as osteochondritis dissecans.

In terms of pathogenesis, it can be considered an area of engorged joint cartilage that is not correctly bound under the subchondral bone (Fig. 10). Tangential force from the scapular may cause this weakened area to rupture vertically. The synovial fluid then reaches the deeper layers of the damaged cartilage, causing synovitis. If no further trauma occurs, the damage may heal. However if trauma continues, the rupture becomes circular and a loose flap is formed inside the joint. This continues to cause synovitis until it is removed.

The cause of the thickening is unknown, although hereditary predisposition is suspected. Feeding with a triple dose of calcium can also cause osteochondrosis.

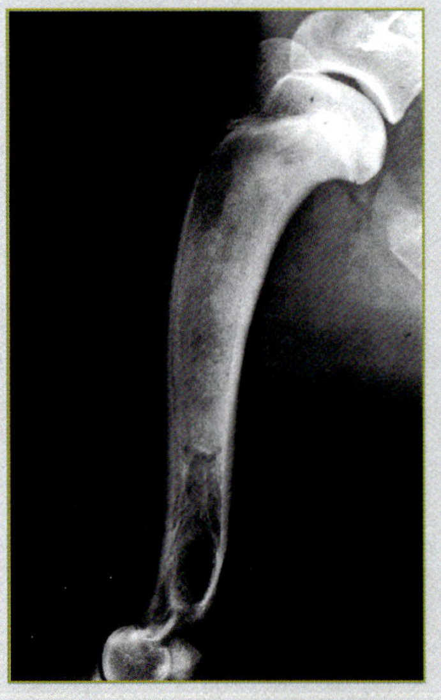

Figure 8. A case of panosteitis, which may lead to a clinically suspected case of OCD, but is easily ruled out by X-ray.

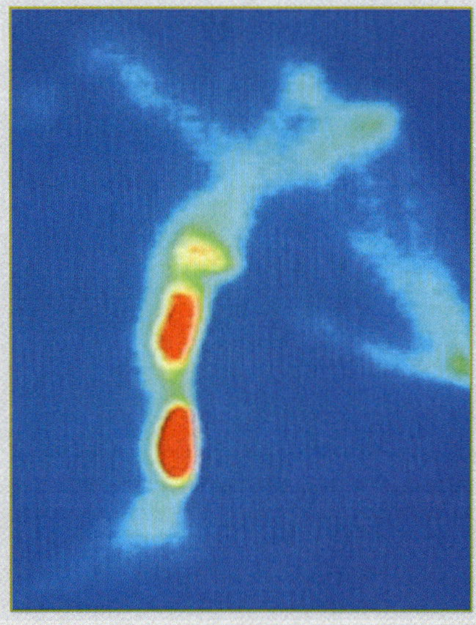

Figure 9. Gammagraphy image of a case of panosteitis. Red denotes the reactive areas, also observed at the humeral head.

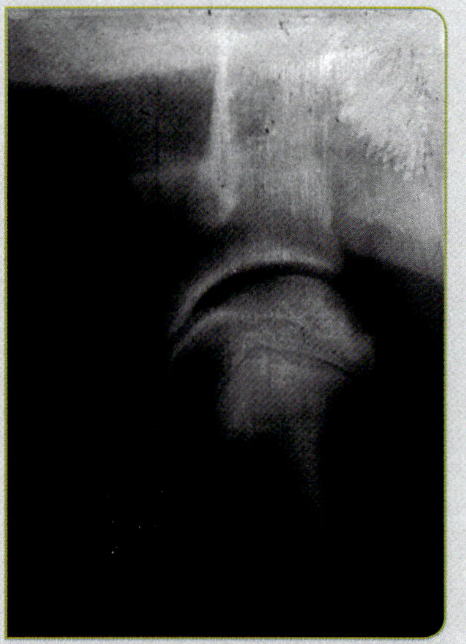

Figure 10. Humeral OCD with radiotransparent image at the caudal area of the affected part.

Optimal growth of large breed puppies

In comparison to other species of animal and humans, as dogs grow, important physical changes take place over a relatively short period of time. Especially in large breeds, long bone growth rate is spectacular. By the age of 16-18 months, these types of dog reach their final body size (although not weight).

Growth cartilage

Bones grow longitudinally through the growth cartilage. Bones do not grow at random; they only grow through the cartilage located at either end. During the growth process, this cartilage becomes mineralised and transforms into bone. The process continues until the bone has reached its final length.

Any abnormalities in this process can lead to skeletal diseases causing lameness and bone deformities. The shoulder and elbow joints tend to be the most commonly affected. The patella (stifle), the hock (tarsus) and the hip joint can also be affected.

Skeletal problems

Research conducted with large breeds of dog in Sweden, the US, Germany, Australia and the Netherlands has shown that these conditions are due to abnormal development of joint cartilage. In dogs, the condition is known as osteochondrosis (OC) or osteochondritis dissecans (OCD). Furthermore, excess load on the joints in overweight animals may also cause problems, the most obvious example of which is hip dysplasia (HD).

OC and HD are conditions that develop in growing puppies. They are hereditary diseases, but can also be influenced by external factors such as trauma. HD is characterised by a poorly fitting hip joint, either due to the shape of the apophysis, the fossa, or both. If a dog does not present HD once its skeleton has matured, it will never suffer from this condition. If the animal suffers from HD but was not diagnosed as a puppy, a diagnosis may be made at a later stage, as a result of subsequent osteoarthritis. The same is true of OCD.

Several studies have proven (excluding genetic factors) that relative excess weight caused by overfeeding in puppies during the growth period (the puppy is overweight for its age in relation to its size) significantly increases the chances of suffering clinical HD. There are important advantages in keeping a puppy's weight under control, and from an orthopaedic perspective, a slim puppy is preferable to an obese puppy. Excess weight causes deformities in the hip joint, and increases the risk of HD. Overall size (height to the withers) is not affected by controlling a puppy's weight. The puppy does not grow more slowly in terms of size, but only in terms of weight gain, which is preferable.

Nutrition as a key factor

The risks of excess calcium intake

Calcium is necessary for the development of healthy bone tissue. Extensive research has shown calcium intake is a major risk factor for the development of OCD. Excess calcium intake increases the risk of the dog developing clinical problems.

This can occur when calcium supplements are added to a full balanced diet, when the animal is fed a complete food with a high calcium content, or when the owner adds too much calcium to "home-made" food. Adding calcium to a full and balanced diet should always be avoided. The amount of calcium contained in these feeds has been calculated carefully.

The dangers of a high calorie diet

No connection has been made between HD and the longitudinal growth of the bones; however, it is strongly affected by nutrition. A high calorie intake during the growth stage carries the risk of developing HD. The mechanism by which this risk increases appears to be due to the rapid increase in weight in turn supported by a relatively immature skeleton.

At birth, the skeleton is fundamentally made of cartilage, which gradually transforms into bone. Unlike bone, cartilage is flexible and can change shape; indeed it does so if subjected to strong loads. When an immature skeleton is "overloaded" due to excess weight for the puppy's age, the hip joint is at risk of changing shape and becoming dysplastic.

However, HD is a hereditary condition, and when the animal does not carry the genes involved, regardless of age, excess weight will never be the cause of HD. However, it has been demonstrated that when there is a risk of HD in the genetic line, overfeeding of the puppy dramatically increases the frequency and severity of the problem.

This also applies to the relative risk of OCD and the combination of disorders known as elbow dysplasia. An excessively fast increase in bodyweight increases the risk of these disorders appearing. In order to obtain the best end result - a healthy dog of the correct size - a balanced growth rate and a steady increase in bodyweight is necessary. Correct feeding ensures that the dog reaches the appropriate adult size and optimum state of health.

The amount of proteins has no effect

Research into the growth of the Great Dane (Nap RC, the Netherlands) has shown that the amount of protein in the diet does not have a significant effect on skeletal development. Feeding a high protein diet does not increase the risk of OCD or HD and has no effect on the longitudinal growth of the bone.

Special food for growth

Despite the high occurrence of bone disorders in large breeds, the good news is that there are specially formulated foods that meet the requirements of rapid growth in large breed puppies. These food are based on recent research that considers calcium to be the main risk factor in food for large breeds, and that also recommend a low calorie diet in order to control the growth rate of these animals.

Diagnosis and treatment

Cartilage cannot normally be seen on X-ray, except where there is dystrophic calcification or bone formation. As OCD lesions consist of the formation of areas of thicker cartilage, a flattened area can be observed. Arthrography is not normally necessary to confirm the diagnosis.

If an early diagnosis is made (between 4-6 months), sometimes conservative treatment is effective (Fig. 11). This consist of rest and low calorie food intake with no calcium supplements. Rest can prevent the formation of cartilage flaps. This is important, as once a flap has formed the injury will not heal. Flaps usually form at the age of 6 months; for this reason dogs that continue to be lame after six and a half months are candidates for surgery.

The cartilage flap usually remains connected to the normal cartilage along the cranial border. If it becomes detached, it remains inside the joint at the caudoventral base of the joint capsule.

Some loose fragments inside the joint can be reabsorbed, some remain viable and others even increase in size as they receive nutrition from the synovial fluid. Others adhere to the synovial membrane, become vasculated and gradually ossifying. These fragments are known as "ossicles". Fragments that migrate to the synovial sheath of the bicipital tendon result in severe lameness.

Male dogs are more commonly affected than females and generally present the condition bilaterally.

Lameness is often observed at late stages (8 months). In these cases either the owners have ignored the symptoms or the veterinary doctors have failed to diagnose the condition in the early stages. Initial lameness is sometimes dismissed as "strong growing pains". Pain during palpation is variable and generally more intense during extreme extension of the the limb than upon flexion or rotation. Crepitation is uncommon and muscular atrophy is evident. The clinical signs are more evident after resting after intense exercise.

The purpose of surgery is to remove the cartilage flap or joint growth that is irritating the synovial membrane, thus smoothing the joint surfaces. The second objective is to remove peripheral cartilage around the lesion not adhered to the underlying tissue. A third consideration is whether to perform curettage or not.

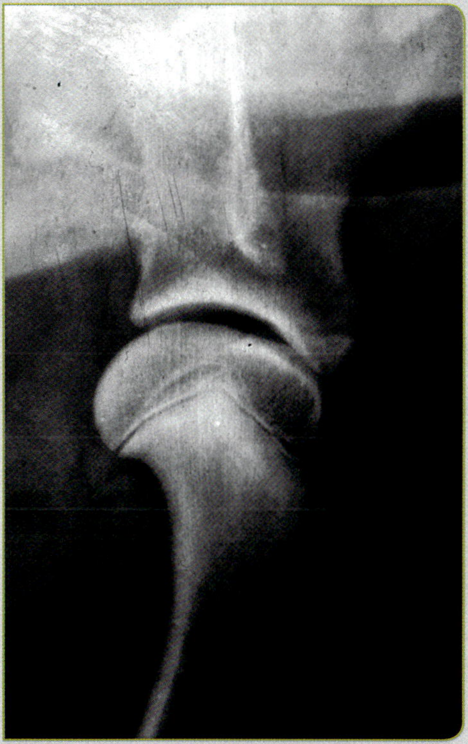

Figure 11. Image with areas of cartilage hypertrophy that together with the clinical details of the animal lead to a suspected diagnosis of OCD, which in this case may response to conservative nutritional treatment.

Curettage is recommended because the granulation tissue of the haemorrhagic subchondral bone invades the fault and swiftly refills it with fibrocartilage. This is the case if the fault is covered by dense sclerotic bone. The defect is often covered by a slightly grey layer (calcified cartilage) which may stimulate healing; if this is the case then curettage may not be necessary.

Another alternative is to make small holes in the damaged in order to allow the vasculature to reform without damaging the existing cartilaginous elements. These vascular channels in the subchondral bone accelerate the growth of the repair tissue in the cartilage defect. This is the authors' preferred technique. As this procedure cannot be effectively performed by arthroscopy, it is preferable to expose the joint.

The surgical approach used is variable. A caudolateral approach, or variants of this is effective if surgery is performed with an assistant. When working alone it is more advisable to perform an osteotomy of the acromion. However, this involves a more lengthy post-operative recovery period.

The caudal base of the joint cavity must always be thoroughly examined for fragments of cartilage. This area can be more easily exposed using a Hohmann separator, with the shoulder and the elbow in flexion.

If fragments of cartilage are observed in the bicipital tendon sheath, a craniomedial approach is required.

The most common complication of this procedure is seroma formation. Seromas can be prevented with postoperative rest for 10-14 days and meticulous suturing of the joint capsule.

03 Calcification of the supraspinatus tendon

This degenerative disease, which causes mild to moderate lameness, has been observed by the authors particularly in the Rottweiler. The aetiology of the condition is unknown, but it is likely to be caused by overuse syndrome. It can occur unilaterally or bilaterally.

Lameness worsens on bearing weight and over the course of the day, lessening with rest. Manipulation of the limb is generally painless.

A special X-ray projection can be used to identify the calcification. It should be remembered that these calcifications are often asymptomatic. Other conditions such as bicipital tendinitis and other chronic joint injuries should be ruled out. The grade and extent of the calcification are not directly proportional to the level of pain experienced by the dog.

Treatment

Treatment consists of a longitudinal incision in the supraspinatus tendon. This is performed with the animal in dorsal recumbency with the forearms strapped to the body. After making the incision through the skin and subcutaneous tissue a deep section is made into the longitudinal fibres of the brachiocephalic muscle. After identifying the supraspinatus muscle tendon, longitudinal incisions are made along the humerus. The calcified matter is white in colour, similar to that observed in case of a calcified disc. The wound is closed in layers.

Post-operative treatment consists of strapping with a flexed carpal for 14 days in order to allow the tendon to heal. Exercise should be limited for 4 weeks.

04

Tenosynovitis of biceps brachii muscle tendon

This muscle tendon originates at the supraglenoid apophysis, running through the intertubercular groove of the humerus where it is supported by the transverse humeral ligament. Finally the tendon inserts into the radius and ulna; its function is elbow flexion. It is encased in a synovial sheath, dependant on the glenohumeral joint capsule. This sheath extends distally beyond the transverse humeral ligament.

The injury is cause by distension of the biceps brachii tendon. The mechanism of the injury may be direct or indirect trauma, or simply overloading the joint. The effect on the tendon as a result of this situation can differ; there may be a laceration of the tendon (Fig. 12), chronic inflammatory processes, or occasionally calcifications. These pathological changes may also be caused by other joint conditions such as osteochondritis dissecans, where joint mice (fragments) migrate towards to the joint sheath resulting in acute synovitis. The proliferation of fibrous connective tissue with adherences between the tendon and the synovial sheath restricts movements and cause pain, with different degrees of lameness.

In general, lameness is aggravated with exercise and there is notable muscular atrophy. Pain in the shoulder joint is not a constant sign, particularly in chronic cases. It can be induced by exerting pressure with a finger on the tendon in the area of the intertubercular groove, while flexing the shoulder and extending the elbow.

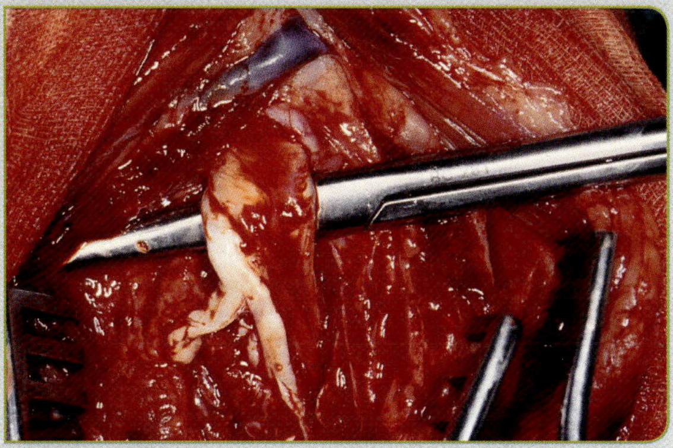

Figure 12. Image of the surgical examination of the biceps tendon, showing a partial tear.

X-ray observations are secondary; there may be bone anomalies at the supraglenoid tuberosity, calcifications on the tendon or osteophytes in the intertubercular groove.

Diagnosis can be facilitated using ultrasound.

Treatment

Conservative treatment consists of antiinflammatory medication, with a strict 8 week confinement period, to reduce the inflammation of the affected structures before the pathological changes become irreversible. A premature return to normal activity will lead to a chronic condition.

This conservative treatment is successful provided there are no pronounced joint mice or osteophytes irritating the tendon. In these cases surgery is generally more effective. The objective of surgery is to remove the friction on the tendon and the inflamed sheath. This is achieved by performing a tenodesis of the bicipital tendon.

This procedure is performed using a craniomedial approach, sectioning the transverse humeral ligament and the joint capsule to access the biceps muscle tendon. The intertubercular groove often presents osteophytes along its borders, and it is therefore advisable to check this area carefully. The tendon is then sectioned close to the supraglenoid tuberosity and attached to the humerus using a screw and washer. Some surgeons prefer to pass the tendon through a bone channel prior to re-attachment, although this is not generally necessary.

Recent reports suggest that arthroscopic sectioning of the tendon is sufficient, without the need to secure it.

This condition often cannot be clearly differentiated from a complete tear of the biceps brachii muscle tendon (Figs. 13 and 14). In cases where lameness does not respond to antiinflammatory treatment and where there is intense pain on palpation, surgical examination of the tendon is recommended.

Postoperative treatment consists of absolute rest for a 4 week period, followed by a gradual return to normal activity.

In cases treated early, recovery is more favourable than in cases where lameness has been present for several months.

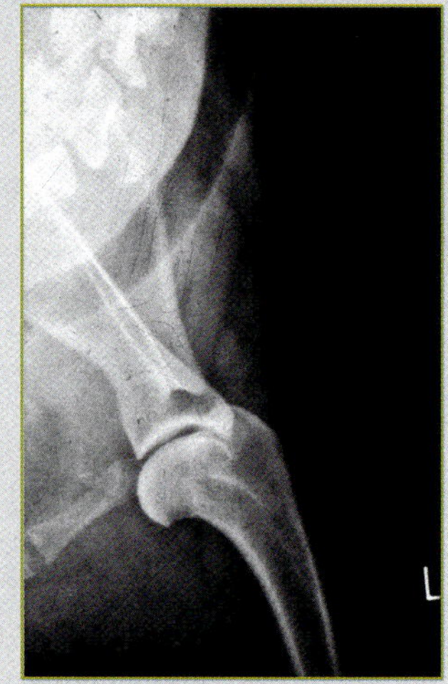

Figure 13. X-ray image of a dog with a healthy biceps brachii muscle tendon.

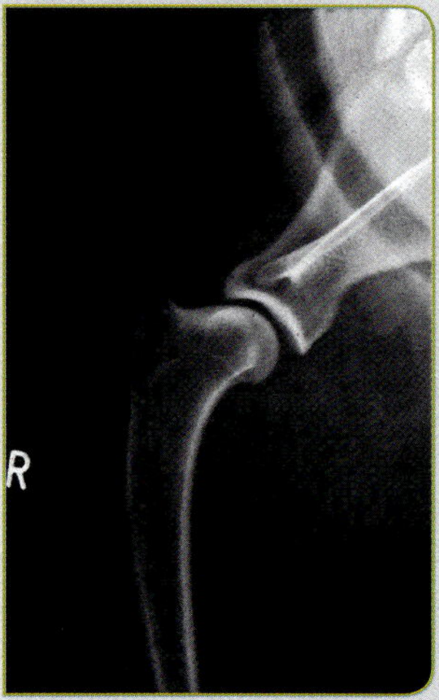

Figure 14. X-ray image of the ruptured tendon. There is anterior displacement of the humerus due to biceps brachii tendon failure.

RSI syndrome

Tenosynovitis of the biceps brachii muscle tendon can be considered to fall under the syndrome known as RSI (Repetitive Strain Injury). Thousands of repetitive movements made over time can cause orthopaedic problems characterised by a loss of muscular strength and sensitivity, pain during movement and at rest, myalgia (muscle pain), tendinitis, tenosynovitis, epicondylitis, tunnel syndrome, peritendinitis, tendomyopathy or insertion desmopathy.

The two main problems affecting the tendons are tendinitis and tenosynovitis. Tendinitis, or the inflammation of a tendon, can affect any tendon, although in dogs it occurs most commonly in the shoulder joint. Tenosynovitis is the inflammation of the tendon sheath surrounding the tendon.

Normally it is the sheath that becomes inflamed, but inflammation may occur in both the sheath and the tendon itself. The cause of tenosynovitis is often unknown, although strain, overuse or excess exercise are generally an influencing factor. In human medicine, tendinitis may also be connected to an illness (for example diabetes or rheumatoid arthritis). Although these correlations have not as yet been published, it is advisable to bear them in mind.

The most common symptoms of tendinitis are:

- Pain upon movement of the tendon.
- Swelling caused by accumulation of fluid and inflammation of the joint.
- Positive biceps test.

A diagnosis of tendinitis can usually be made based on a physical examination and full medical records. A diagnosis is usually confirmed after completing some further tests in order to exclude other possible conditions or illnesses. An analysis of the articular fluid can help to exclude infection, while X-rays can exclude OCD.

Diagnostic imaging techniques

The following are pairs of images comparing transparent plastinated sections of real structures compared with images obtained using CAT and MRI.

Transparent plastinated sections + CAT

SAGITTAL SECTION OF THE SHOULDER JOINT IN EXTENSION

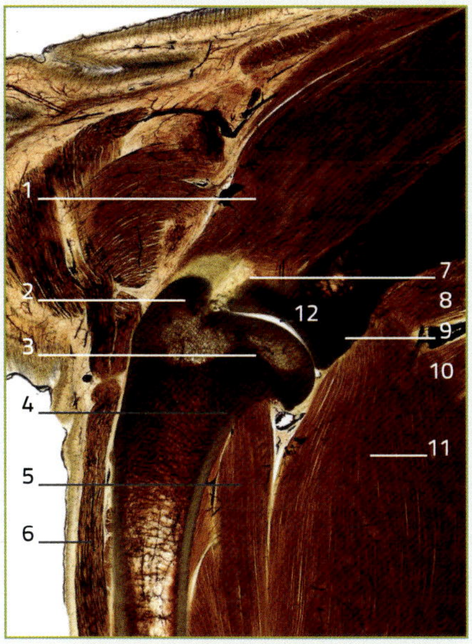

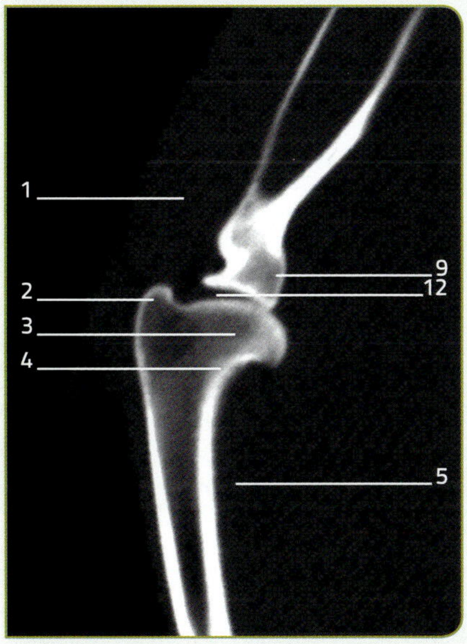

1	Supraspinatus muscle
2	Greater tubercle
3	Head of humerus
4	Neck of humerus
5	Triceps brachii muscle, medial head
6	Cleidobrachialis muscle
7	Supraglenoid tubercle
8	Teres major muscle
9	Infraglenoid tubercle
10	Latissimus dorsi muscle
11	Triceps brachii muscle, long head
12	Glenoid cavity of the scapula

TRANSVERSAL SECTION OF THE SHOULDER JOINT IN EXTENSION

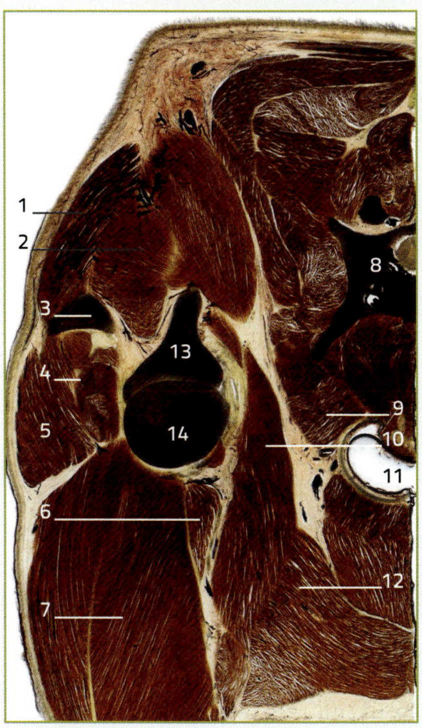

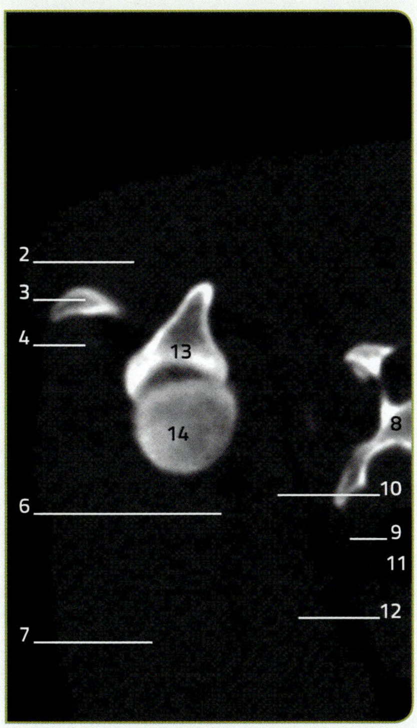

1	Omotransversarius muscle
2	Supraspinatus muscle
3	Acromion
4	Infraspinatus muscle
5	Deltoid muscle
6	Coracobrachialis muscle
7	Triceps brachii muscle
8	Cervical vertebra
9	Longus capitis muscle
10	Deep pectoral muscle
11	Trachea
12	Superficial pectoral muscle
13	Scapula, glenoid cavity
14	Head of humerus

Transparent plastinated sections + MRI

SAGITTAL SECTION OF THE SHOULDER JOINT IN EXTENSION

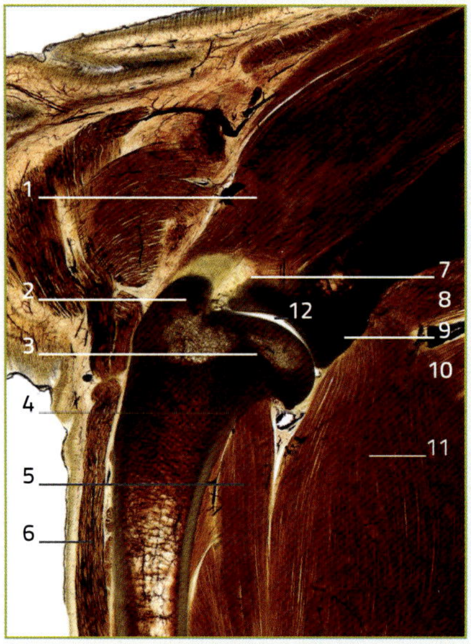

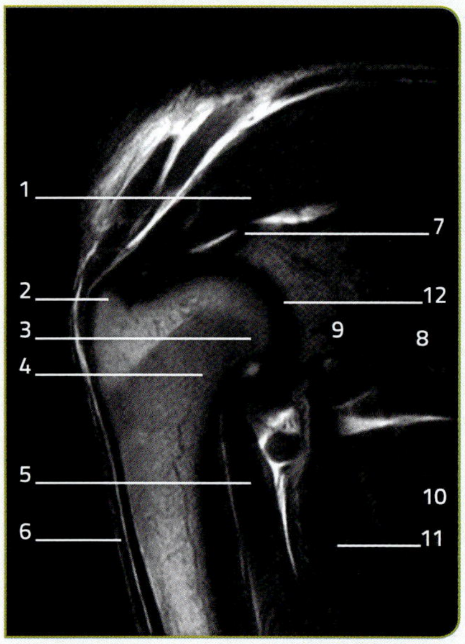

1	Supraspinatus muscle
2	Greater tubercle
3	Head of humerus
4	Neck of humerus
5	Triceps brachii muscle, medial head
6	Cleidobrachialis muscle
7	Supraglenoid tubercle
8	Teres major muscle
9	Infraglenoid tubercle
10	Latissimus dorsi muscle
11	Triceps brachii muscle, long head
12	Glenoid cavity of the scapula

TRANSVERSAL SECTION OF THE SHOULDER JOINT IN EXTENSION

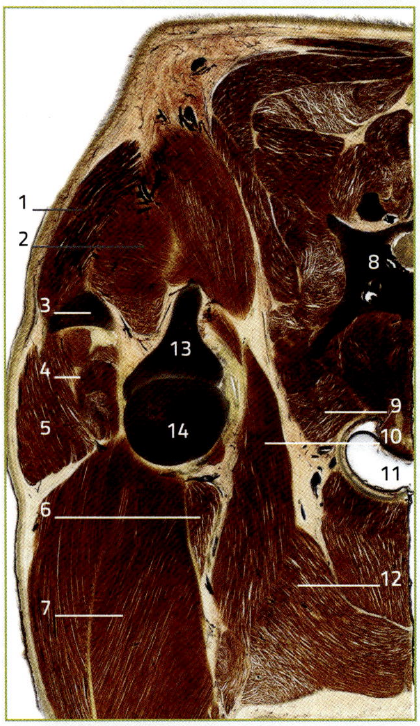

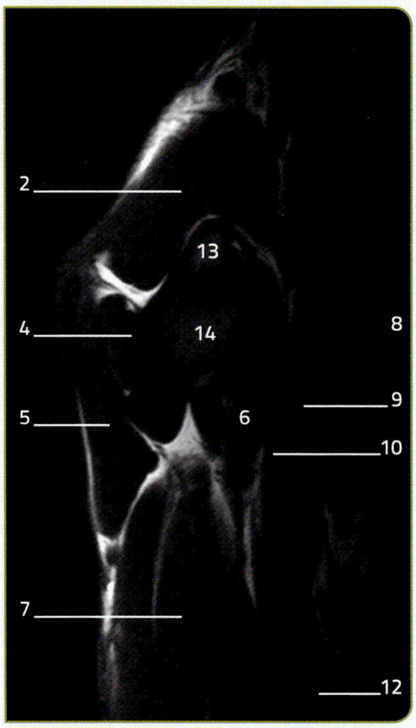

1	Omotransversarius muscle
2	Supraspinatus muscle
3	Acromion
4	Infraspinatus muscle
5	Deltoid muscle
6	Coracobrachialis muscle
7	Triceps brachii muscle
8	Cervical vertebra
9	Longus capitis muscle
10	Deep pectoral muscle
11	Trachea
12	Superficial pectoral muscle
13	Scapula, glenoid cavity
14	Head of humerus

SURGICAL APPROACHES

Approach to the craniolateral region of the shoulder joint via tenotomy of the infraspinatus muscle

1 The skin incision extends from the greater tubercle towards the lateral humeral epicondyle. The course of the cephalic vein should be avoided although, as with the omobrachial vein, a ligature can be made if necessary.

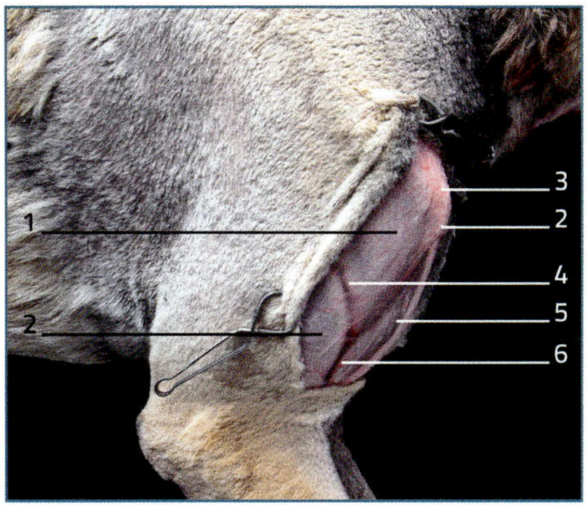

1 Acromial portion of deltoid muscle
2 Omobrachial fascia
3 Greater tubercle of the humerus
4 Axillobrachial vein
5 Brachiocephalic muscle
6 Cephalic vein

2 The acromial portion of the deltoid muscle must be released. The cranial border is taken as a reference point for caudal displacement.

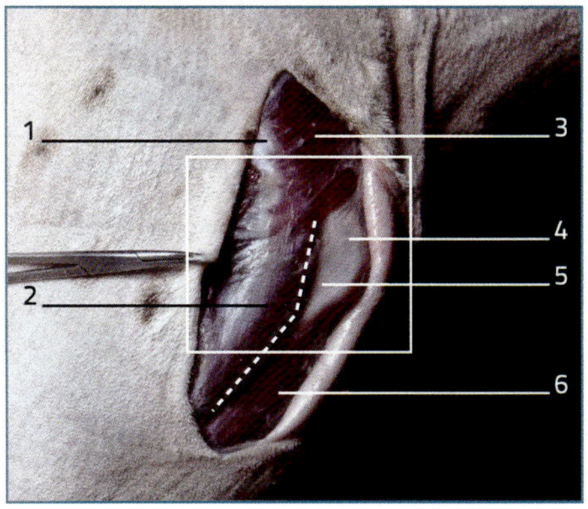

1 Acromion
2 Acromial portion of deltoid muscle
3 Omotransversarius muscle
4 Greater tubercle of the humerus
5 Omobrachial fascia
6 Brachiocephalic muscle

3 After caudally displacing the acromial portion of the deltoid muscle, the teres minor muscle is located, together with the tendon of insertion of the infraspinatus muscle. The tenotomy is then performed at the points indicated.

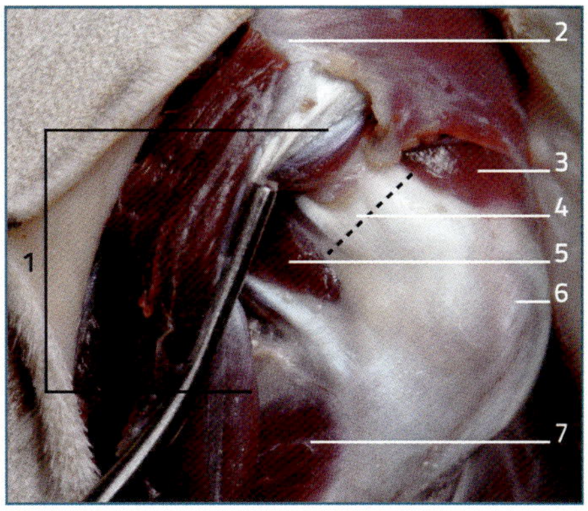

1 Acromial portion of deltoid muscle
2 Acromion
3 Supraspinatus muscle
4 Tendon of the infraspinatus muscle
5 Teres minor muscle
6 Greater tubercle of the humerus
7 Brachial muscle

4 The tendon of insertion of the infraspinatus muscle is displaced dorsally and caudally in order to expose the joint capsule.

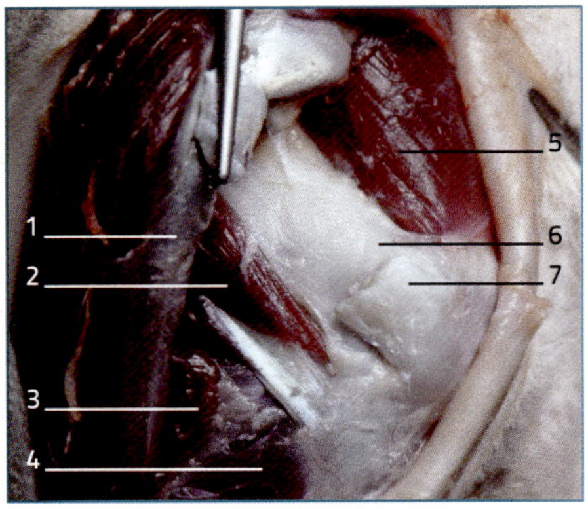

1 Acromial portion of deltoid muscle
2 Teres minor muscle
3 Lateral head of triceps brachii muscle
4 Brachial muscle
5 Supraspinatus muscle
6 Joint capsule
7 Sectioned tendon of the infraspinatus muscle

5 An incision is made into the joint capsule in order to examine the joint surfaces.

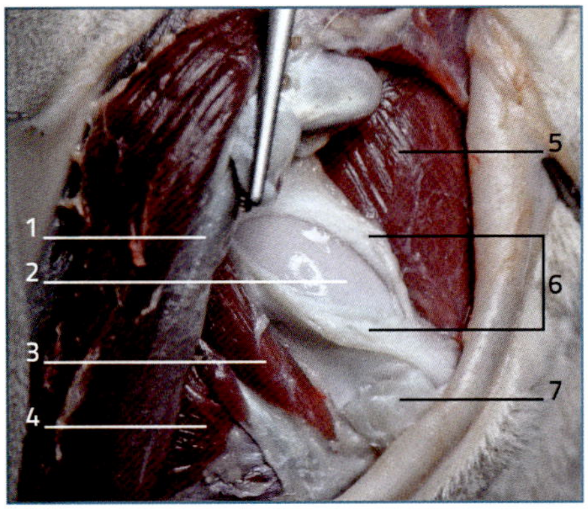

1 Acromial portion of deltoid muscle
2 Head of humerus
3 Teres minor muscle
4 Lateral head of triceps brachii muscle
5 Supraspinatus muscle
6 Joint capsule
7 Sectioned tendon of the infraspinatus muscle

6 The teres minor muscle can be displaced distally for greater exposure of the joint surface. Furthermore, internal rotation of the humerus allows greater exposure of the humeral head.

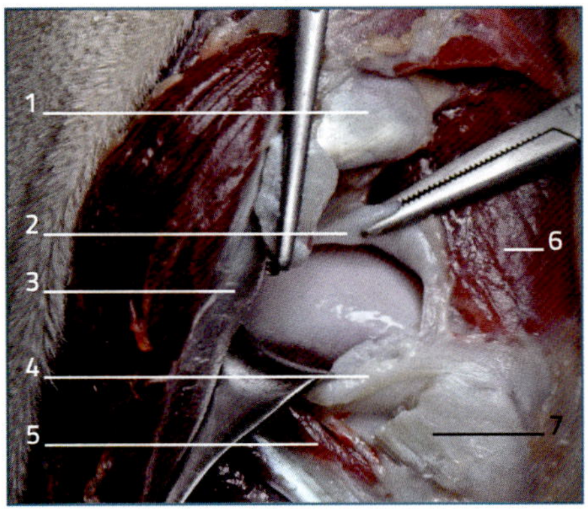

1 Acromion
2 Glenoid lip
3 Acromial portion of deltoid muscle
4 Joint capsule
5 Teres minor muscle
6 Supraspinatus muscle
7 Sectioned tendon of the infraspinatus muscle

Approach to the caudolateral region of the shoulder joint

1 The skin incision runs in a curve from the distal end of the scapular spine to the mid third of the upper arm.

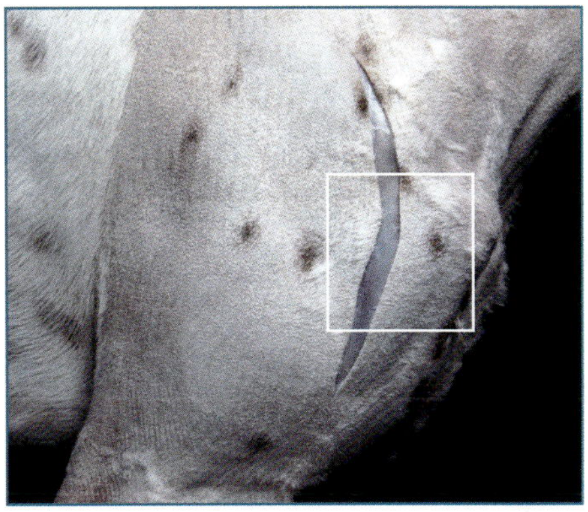

2 After sectioning the omobrachial fascia, a deeper incision must be made between the acromial portion and scapular portion of the deltoid muscle.

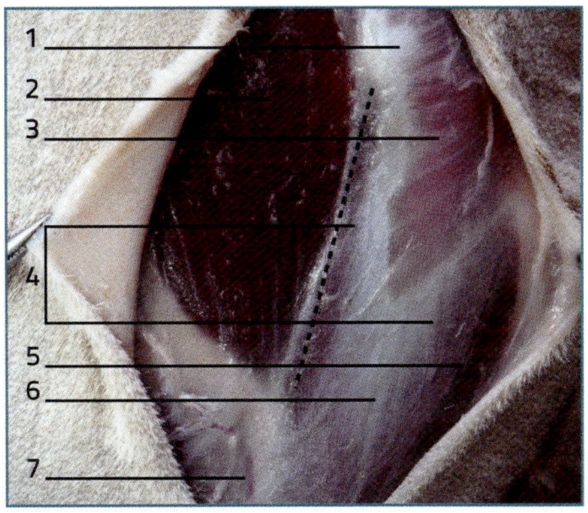

1 Acromion
2 Scapular portion of deltoid muscle
3 Omotransversarius muscle
4 Omobrachial fascia
5 Omobrachial vein
6 Acromial portion of deltoid muscle
7 Axillobrachial vein

3 The two portions of the deltoid muscle are separated to access the joint capsule. The course of the muscular branches of the axillary nerve and the caudal humeral circumflex vessels are then located, as they must not be damaged.

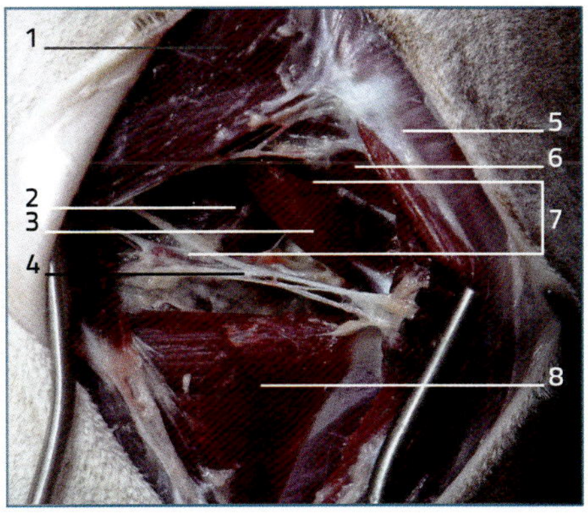

1 Scapular portion of deltoid muscle
2 Long head of triceps brachii muscle
3 Teres minor muscle
4 Muscular branches of the axillary nerve
5 Acromial portion of deltoid muscle
6 Infraspinatus muscle
7 Caudal humeral circumflex artery and vein
8 Lateral head of triceps brachii muscle

4 After sectioning the joint capsule and forcing internal rotation of the humerus, the caudal area of the joint can be freely accessed.

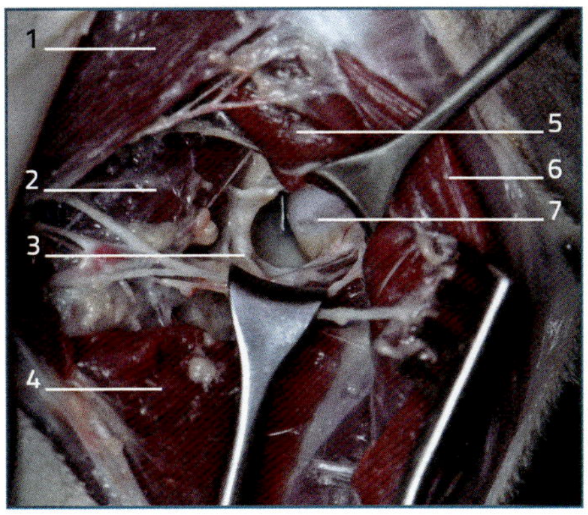

1 Scapular portion of deltoid muscle
2 Long head of triceps brachii muscle
3 Joint capsule
4 Lateral head of triceps brachii muscle
5 Teres minor muscle
6 Acromial portion of deltoid muscle
7 Head of humerus

Approach to the craniomedial region of the shoulder joint

1 The thoracic limb should be placed in abduction, showing the medial surface of the shoulder and upper arm. The skin incision should extend several centimetres proximally and distally to the greater tubercle of the humerus.

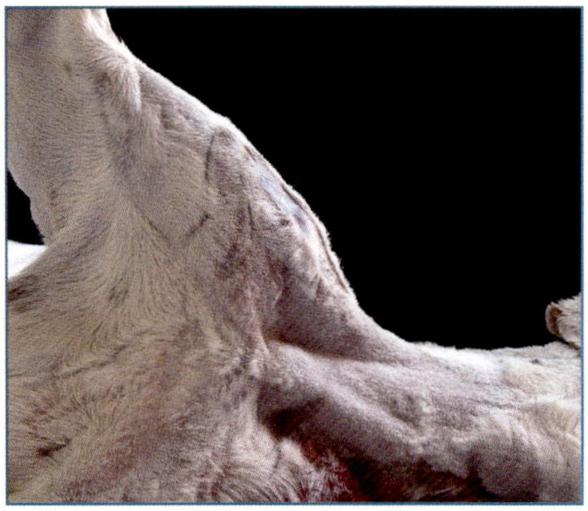

2 After retracting the skin, a deep insertion is made into the space between the brachiocephalic and superficial pectoral muscles.

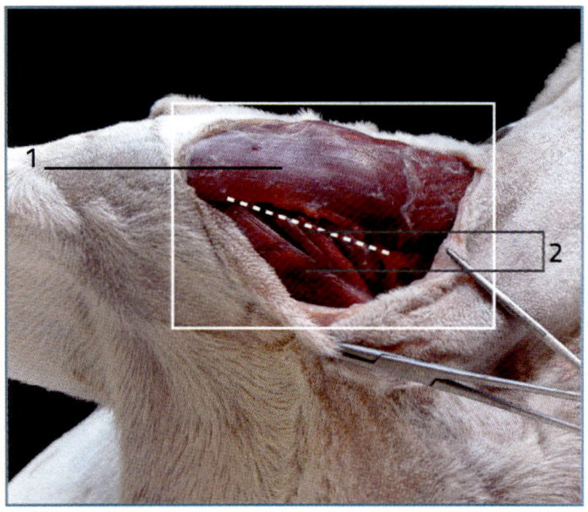

1 Brachiocephalic muscle
2 Superficial pectoral muscle

3 The brachiocephalic muscle is displaced laterally, thus revealing the insertion of the superficial pectoral muscle on the humerus, which must be sectioned.

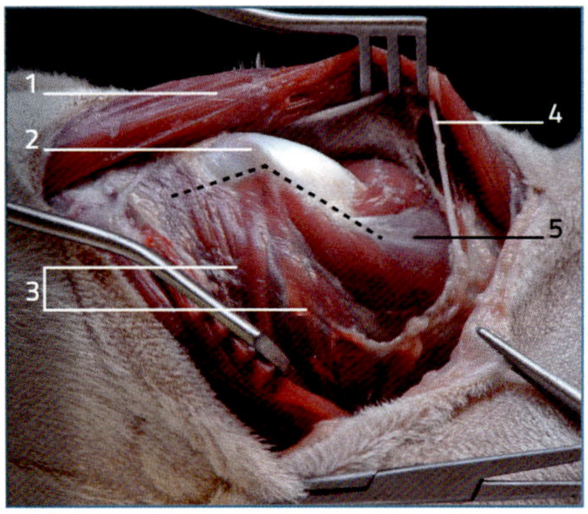

1 Brachiocephalic muscle
2 Greater tubercle of the humerus
3 Superficial pectoral muscle
4 Cephalic vein
5 Supraspinatus muscle

4 The superficial pectoral muscle is displaced medially, showing the insertion of the supraspinatus muscle on the greater tubercle of the humerus and the attachment of the deep pectoral muscle to the humerus, which must be detached in order to gain deeper access to the joint.

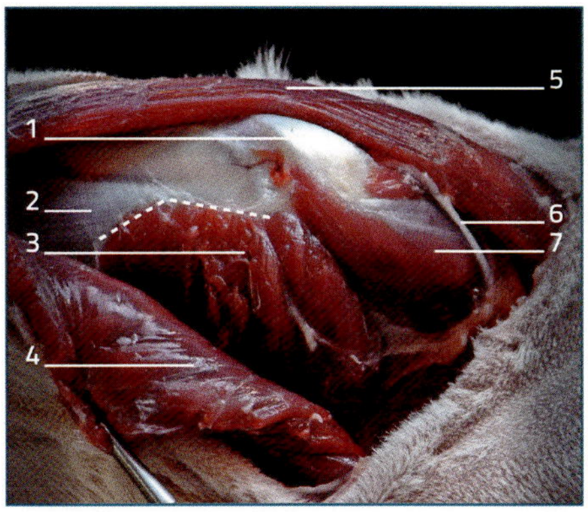

1 Greater tubercle of the humerus
2 Biceps brachii muscle
3 Deep pectoral muscle
4 Superficial pectoral muscle
5 Brachiocephalic muscle
6 Cephalic vein
7 Supraspinatus muscle

5 Once the deep pectoral muscle has been sectioned and displaced medially, the tendons of the subscapularis and coracobrachial muscles are seen over the joint capsule.

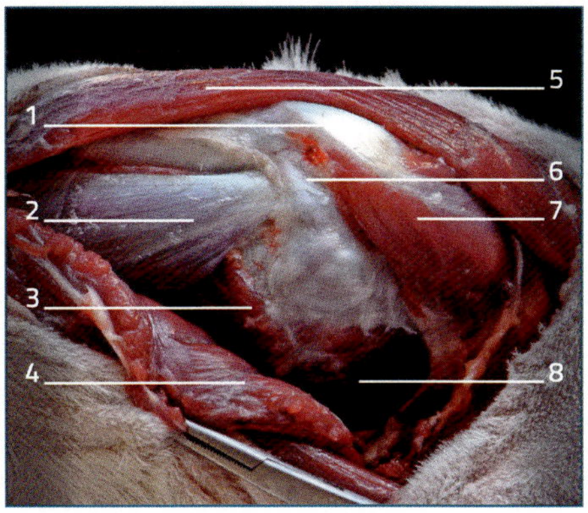

1 Greater tubercle of the humerus
2 Biceps brachii muscle
3 Coracobrachial muscle
4 Deep pectoral muscle
5 Brachiocephalic muscle
6 Transverse ligament of the shoulder joint
7 Supraspinatus muscle
8 Subscapularis muscle

6 The tendon of insertion of the subscapularis muscle and the tendon of origin of the coracobrachial muscle are sectioned to allow medial access to the joint. After opening the capsule the joint cavity and humeral head are exposed.

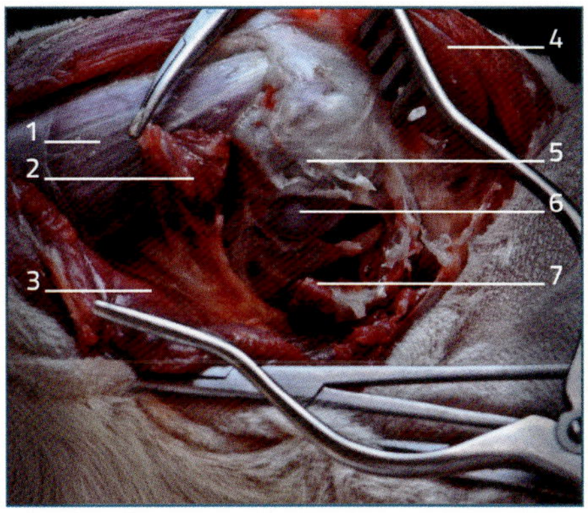

1 Biceps brachii muscle
2 Coracobrachial muscle
3 Deep pectoral muscle
4 Supraspinatus muscle
5 Joint capsule
6 Head of humerus
7 Subscapularis muscle

7 Medial view with external rotation of the humerus to expose the entire joint cavity. Partial detachment of the suprascapular muscle exposes the tendon of the biceps brachii muscle from its origin on the supraglenoid tubercle.

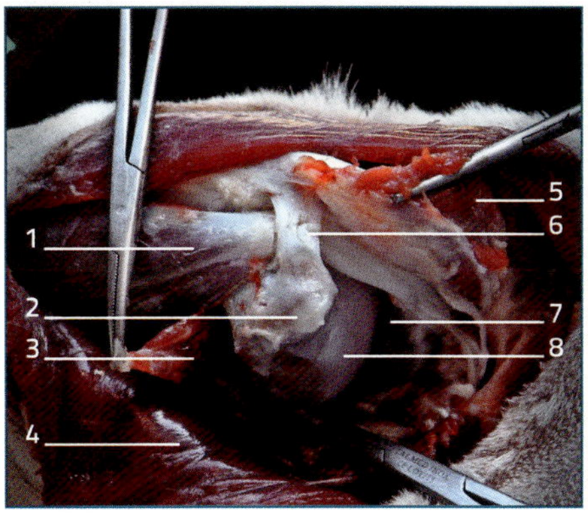

1 Biceps brachii muscle
2 Joint capsule
3 Coracobrachial muscle
4 Deep pectoral muscle
5 Supraspinatus muscle
6 Transverse ligament of the shoulder joint
7 Glenoid cavity
8 Head of humerus

The images included for surgical approaches are adapted from: Latorre, R., Gil, F., Climent, S., López, O., Henry, R., Ayala, M., Ramírez, G., Martínez, F., Vázquez, J.M. *Color Atlas of Surgical Approaches to the Bones and Joints of the Dog and Cat.* Intermédica S.A., 2009; pp. 0-266. ISBN 978-950-555-353-2.

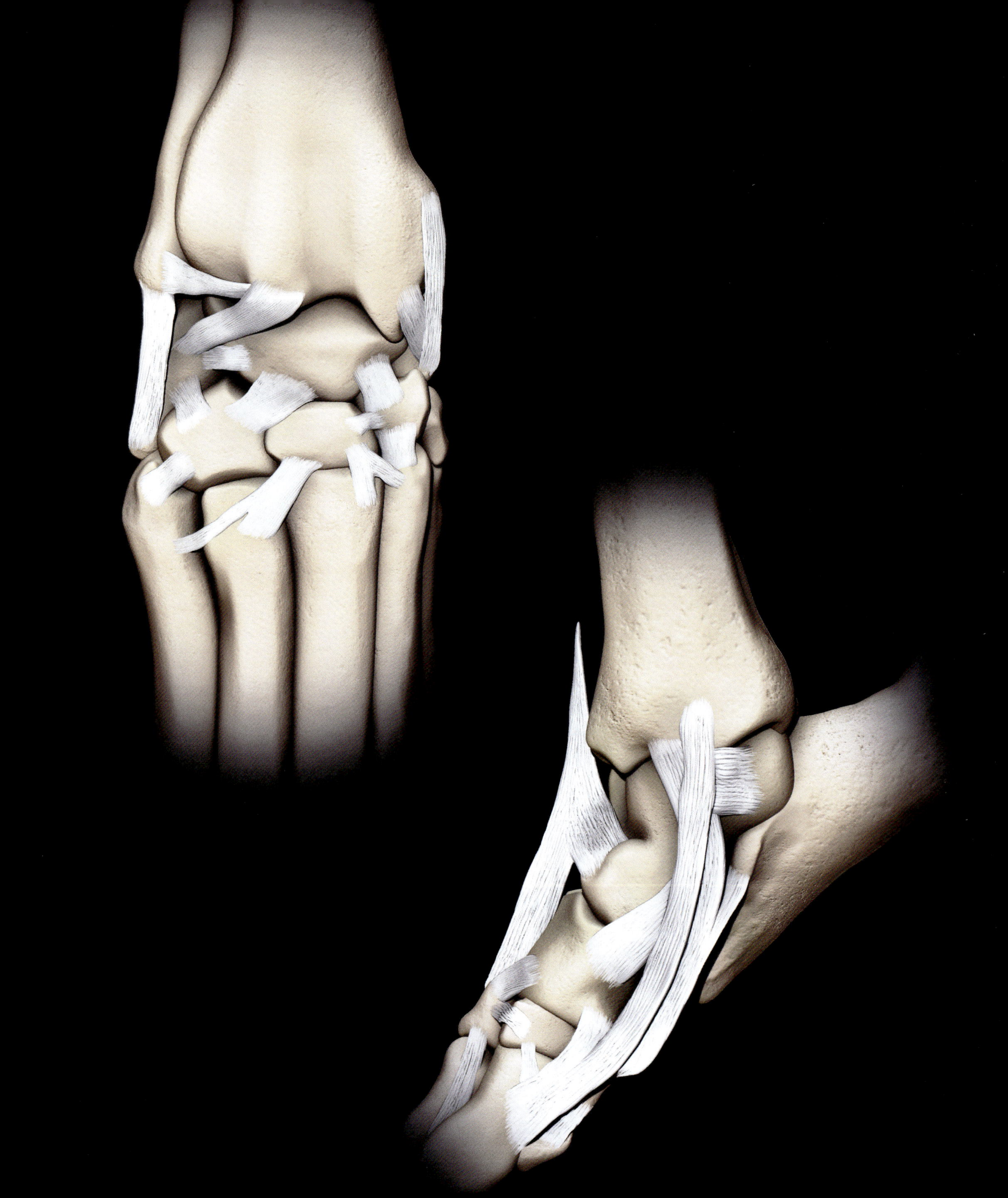

CARPAL AND TARSAL JOINTS

Carpal joint

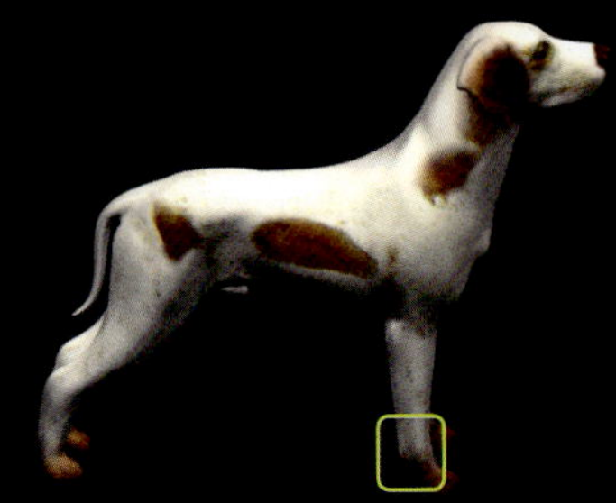

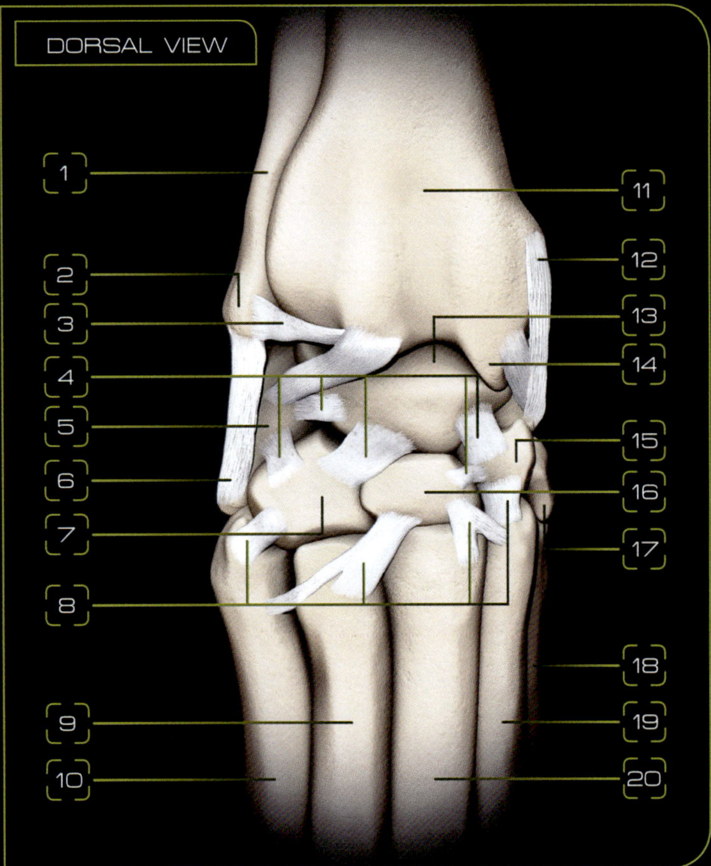

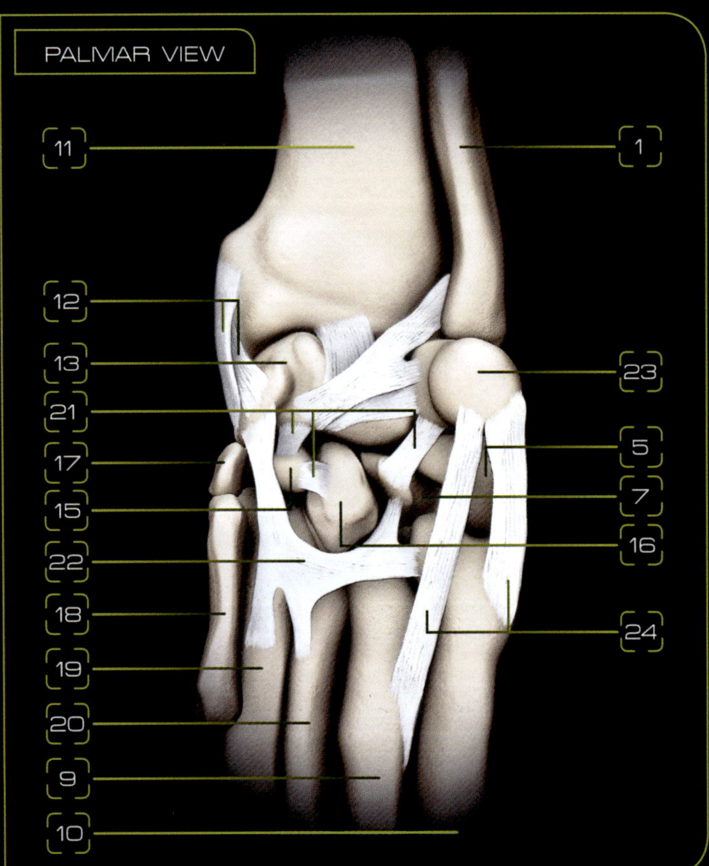

Watch this video on the electronic version
Thoracic limb

Watch this video on the electronic version
Carpal joint and manus

1 Ulna
2 Ulnar styloid apophysis
3 Radioulnar lig.
4 Dorsal intercarpal ligs.
5 Ulnar carpal bone
6 Lateral collateral lig.
7 Fourth carpal bone
8 Dorsal carpometacarpal ligs.
9 Fourth metacarpal bone
10 Fifth metacarpal bone
11 Radius
12 Medial collateral lig.
13 Radial intermediate carpal bone
14 Radial styloid apophysis
15 Second carpal bone
16 Third carpal bone
17 First carpal bone
18 First metacarpal bone
19 Second metacarpal bone
20 Third metacarpal bone
21 Palmar intercarpal ligs.
22 Palmar carpometacarpal ligs.
23 Accessory carpal bone
24 Accessory metacarpal lig.

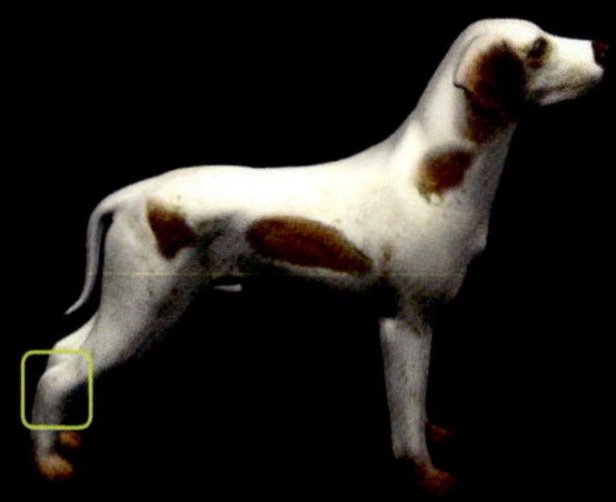

Tarsal joint

Watch this video on the electronic version
Pelvic limb

Watch this video on the electronic version
Tarsus and hind paw

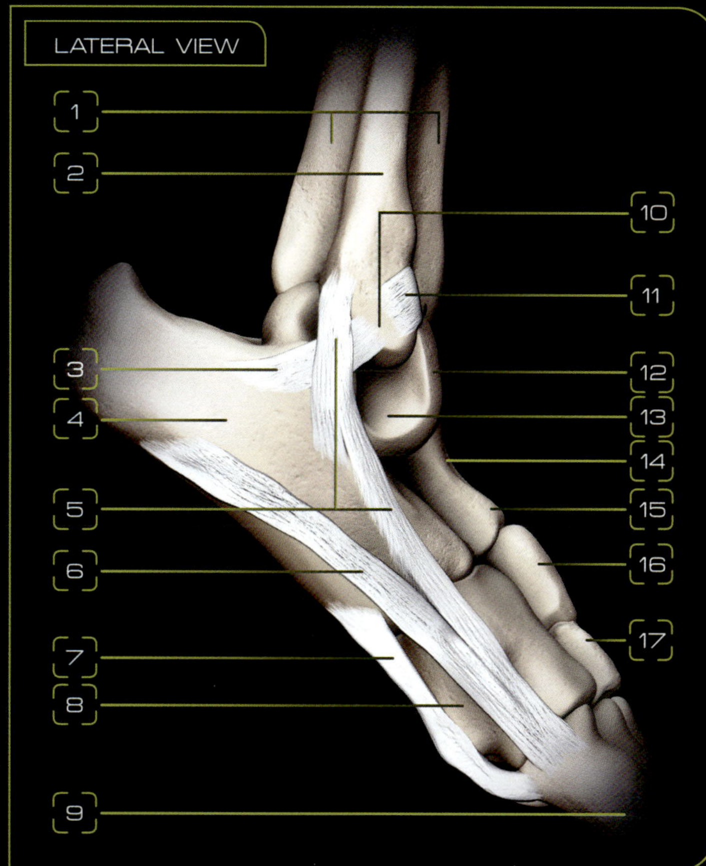

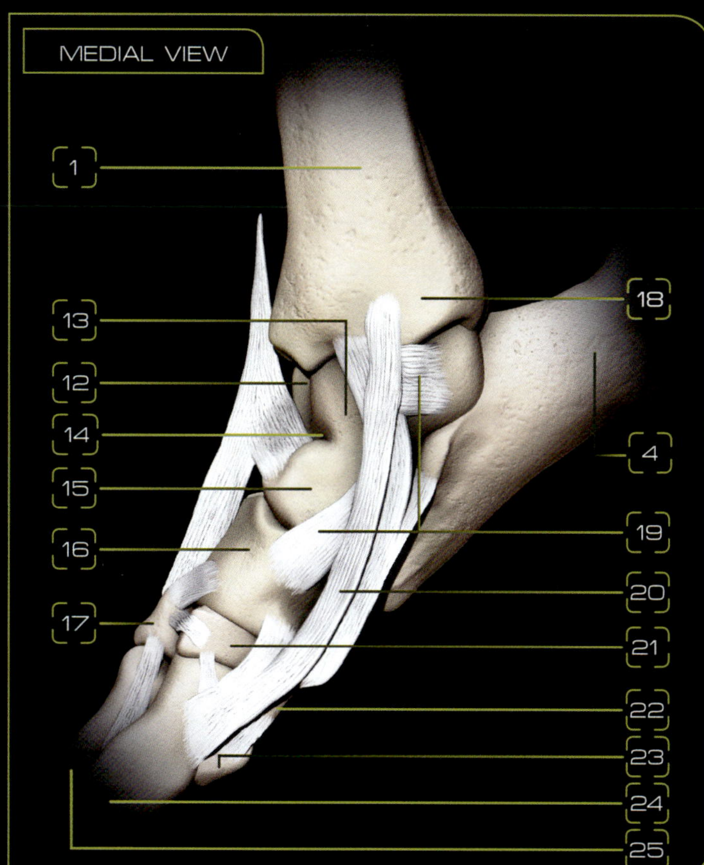

1 Tibia
2 Fibula
3 Lateral collateral lig., short part
4 Calcaneus
5 Lateral collateral lig., long part
6 Abductor muscle of the fifth toe
7 Long plantar lig.
8 Fourth tarsal bone
9 Fifth metatarsal bone
10 Lateral malleolus of the fibula
11 Distal tibiofibular lig.
12 Trochlea of talus bone
13 Body of talus bone
14 Neck of talus bone
15 Head of talus bone
16 Central tarsal bone
17 Third tarsal bone
18 Medial malleolus of the tibia
19 Medial collateral lig., short part
20 Medial collateral lig., long part
21 Second tarsal bone
22 First tarsal bone
23 First metatarsal bone
24 Second metatarsal bone
25 Third metatarsal bone

Orthopaedic conditions of the carpal and tarsal joints

In these joints, the most commonly occurring problems are:

01 Carpal luxation and subluxation: hyperextension

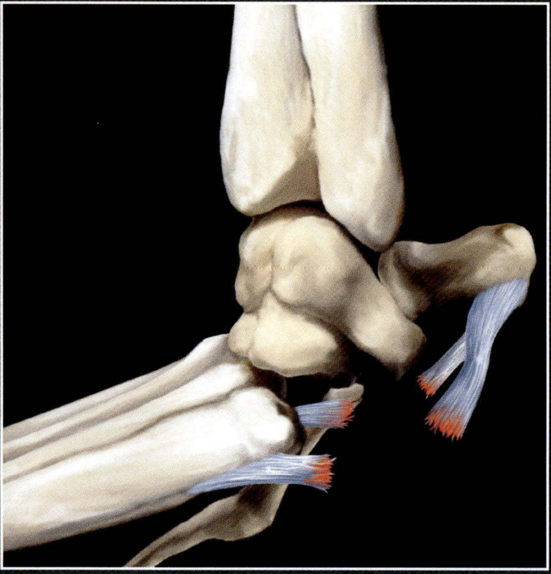

02 Tarsal luxation and subluxation

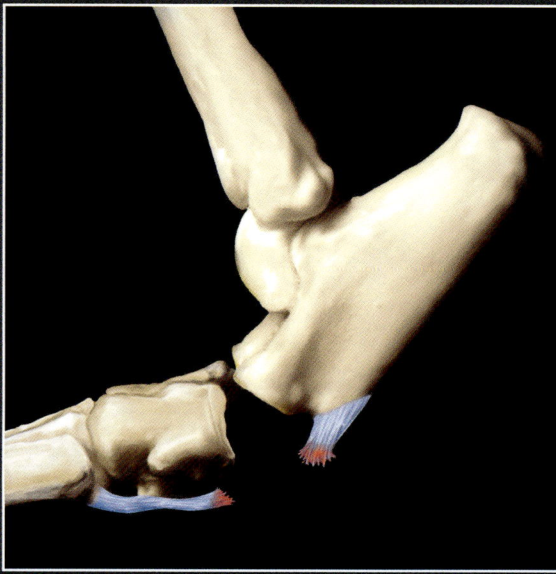

03 Medial tarsal abrasion

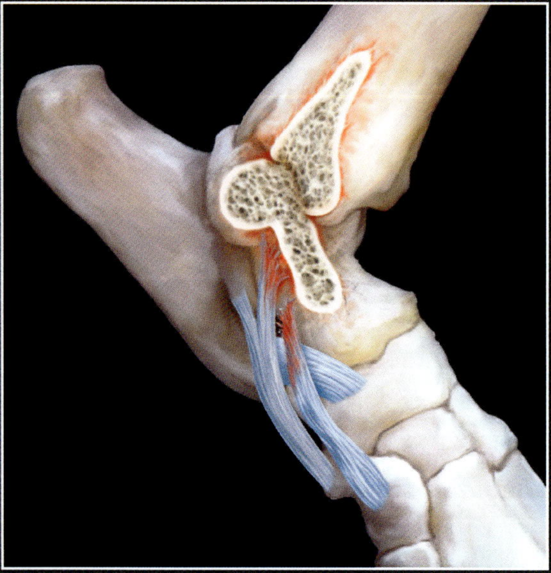

04 Osteochondritis dissecans of the tarsus (talus)

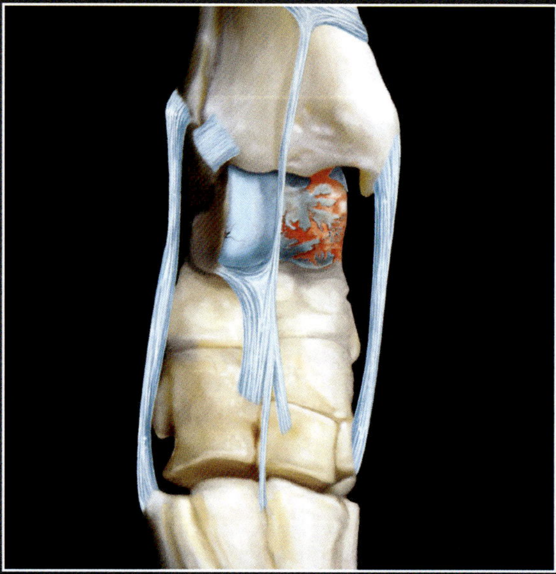

Carpal joint

Given the focus of this book on joint anatomy, the tarsus is perhaps the joint that presents the largest number of problems and to which we will devote more attention. However, in the carpal joint, trauma injuries are the most common cause of lameness in this joint and in the toes. Injury caused by jumping from cars or buildings result in carpal and metacarpal fractures or hyperextension of the joints due to tears in the supporting ligaments and fibrous cartilage.

Gunshot wounds are significant in the carpal joint due to the loss of a large amount of soft tissue - already scarce, and results in joint contamination and the loss of the collateral supporting ligament. Gunshot wounds also present further problems as the cartilage cells are poisoned by lead in the joint, leading to chondrolysis, hypertrophic arthritis and periarticular fibrosis.

Examination of the carpal joint will reveal palpable signs of inflammation and pain. Fractures are more common in the metacarpals than in the metatarsals. Clinical signs depend on the severity of the fracture and degree of displacement. Inflammation of soft tissue may be minimal if the fracture is not displaced or affects only one bone. In chronic carpal fractures, periarticular fibrosis appears similar to a thickening of the joint capsule and is easily detectable alongside the concurrent synovitis. In cases of chronic luxation, the animal will place weight on the limb exacerbating the deformity secondary to the ligament damage. For example, if the medial collateral ligament is damaged, the dog will use the limb in valgus, whereas is the injury is located in the palmar area, the limb will be used in hyperextension. If there are large displaced bone fragments, pain and crepitation will be evident upon manipulating the joint.

Joint effusion is easily detected by palpation on the dorsal side of the joint and may be indicative of osteoarthritis, fractures and ligament rupture or elongation. If the distal part of the radius cannot be easily located with the carpal joint flexed at 90°, there is joint effusion.

A reduction or increase in the range of movement in the carpal joint indicates some kind of structural issue. The range of flexion and extension is examined by keeping the distal part of the forearm steady, and moving the carpal joint in search for signs of pain.

01 Carpal luxation and subluxation: hyperextension

The physiological extension of the carpal joint is limited to 10°; hyperextension suggests a rupture of palmar ligaments or the palmar fibrous cartilage structure (Figs. 1-8). This is one of the most common carpal injuries, and is associate with jumps or falls. Affected animals present grade IV claudication, in particular in the first few days, after which time the claudication gradually diminishes. If the animal is forced to place weight on the limb, there is a notable hyperextension of the carpal joint and, in severe cases, the carpal pad may be touching the the ground. Pronation and supination of the carpal joint are normal when the joint is in flexion, but both movements are limited upon extension. In order to establish normal function of collateral ligaments, medial and lateral tension is applied. The medial (radial) collateral ligament is more commonly damaged than the lateral (ulnar), as it is under continuous stress due to the nature of the standing position in the dog, where the forepaw is held slightly in valgus.

The area of instability is easily located by palpation, and collateral ligament integrity is determined by placing the dog in a forced varus or valgus position. If there is obvious valgus displacement, there is damage to the medial (radial) collateral ligament; in varus, the lateral (ulnar) collateral ligament is affected. The contralateral carpal joint must also be palpated to establish any abnormal displacement.

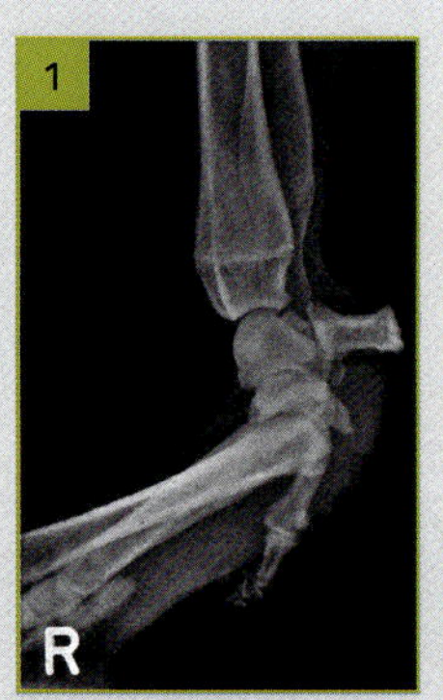

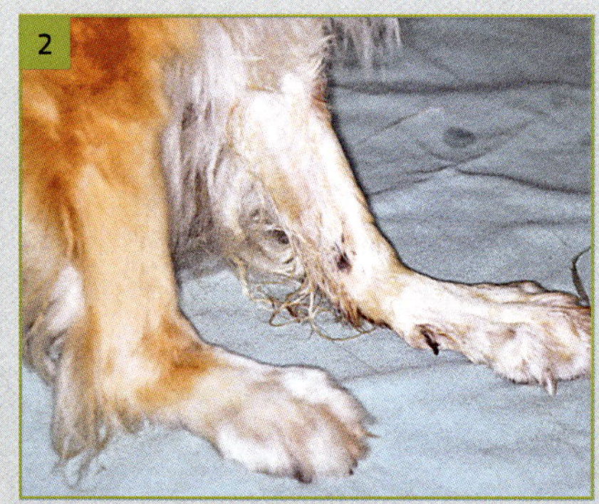
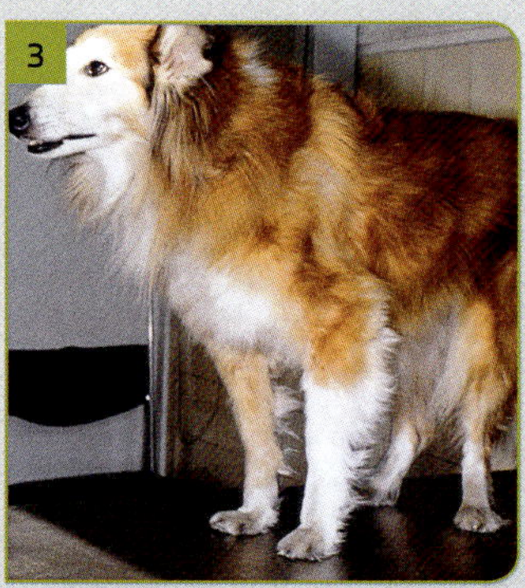
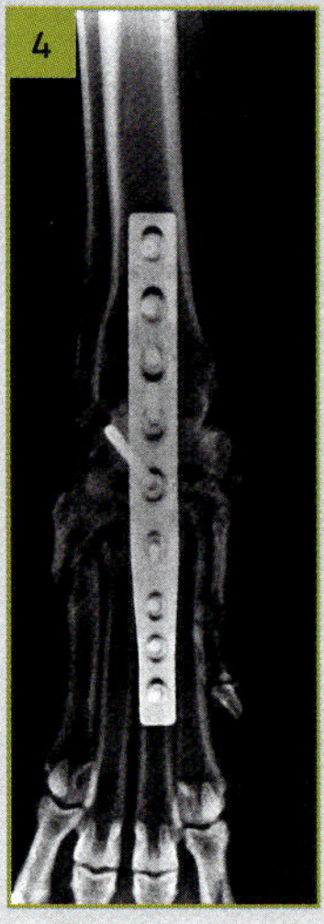
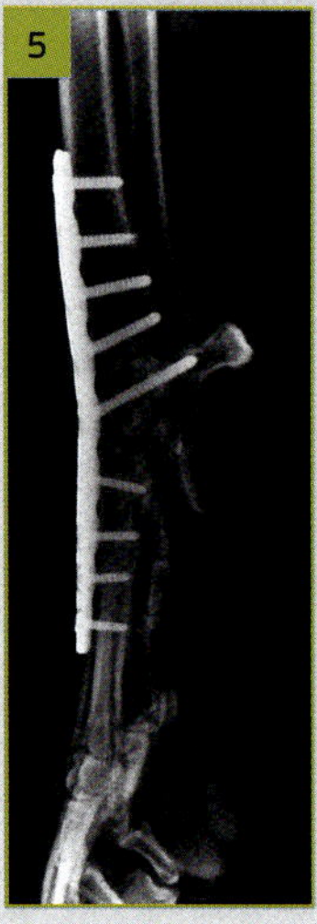
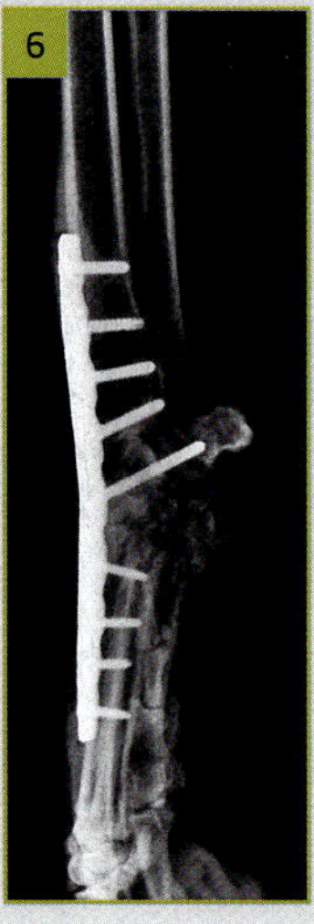
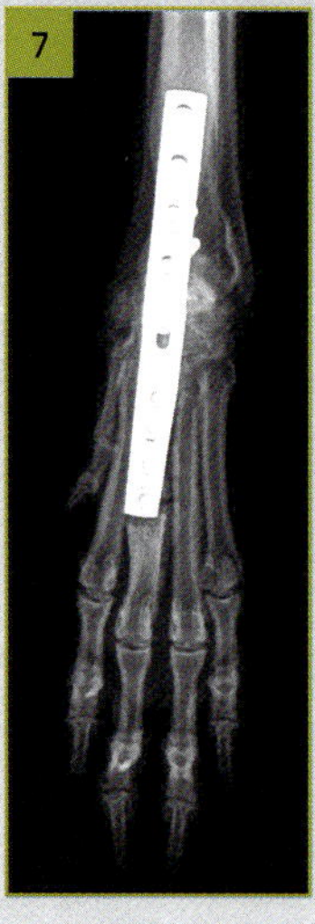
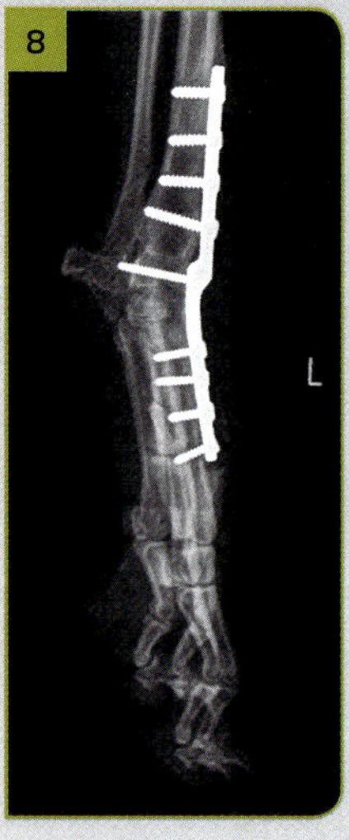

Figure 1. X-ray image of hyperextension of the carpal joint.
Figure 2. A dog with hyperextension in both carpal joints. Here the cause is arthritis of rheumatic origin.
Figure 3. Image of the same dog after bilateral pan-arthrodesis.
Figure 4. X-ray image showing a dorsal plate fitted between the radius and the third metacarpal.
Figure 5. Lateral X-ray image, showing the central screw reaching the accessory carpal.
Figure 6. Lateral X-ray image of the animal, 8 weeks after surgery.
Figure 7. X-ray image of another case. Arthrodesis with a special staggered plate, 8 weeks after surgery.
Figure 8. Laterolateral image of the previous case after the same period.

Tarsal joint

02

Tarsal luxation and subluxation

This section focuses on orthopaedic conditions of the tarsus, as the carpal joint is most commonly affected by trauma induced problems that are resolved with appropriate osteosynthesis or via full or partial arthrodesis. However, the tarsal joint presents a casuistry far richer in orthopaedic problems, and the treatment options described for trauma injuries can be extrapolated to the carpal joint. In any event, and given the general scope of this publication, we will only present a representative sample of joint injuries at this level. The bones affected in the tarsus are the talus, the calcaneus and the central tarsal bone.

Tibiotarsal luxations

Tibiotarsal luxations are associated with the rupture of the collateral ligaments and the joint capsule. The damaged ligaments can be sutured, repositioned on the bone, or replaced with synthetic material.

If there is severe damage to the soft tissue, additional support from a bilateral external fixture is required. In case of fractured malleolus bones, open surgery is required to reduce the luxation and fit a cerclage.

Proximal plantar intertarsal subluxation

Another of the most common pathologies in the tarsus is proximal plantar intertarsal subluxation (rupture of the long plantar ligament or plantare longum) (Fig. 9). In these cases the dog will adopt a plantigrade stance when walking. Diagnosis is made primarily via physical examination, and treatment consists of partial arthrodesis of the joint. A tension band and a Steinmann pin are fitting from the tuber calcanei through the fourth tarsal bone and third metatarsal bone (Figs. 10 and 11), between the first and fourth metatarsals, or between the fourth and fifth metatarsals.

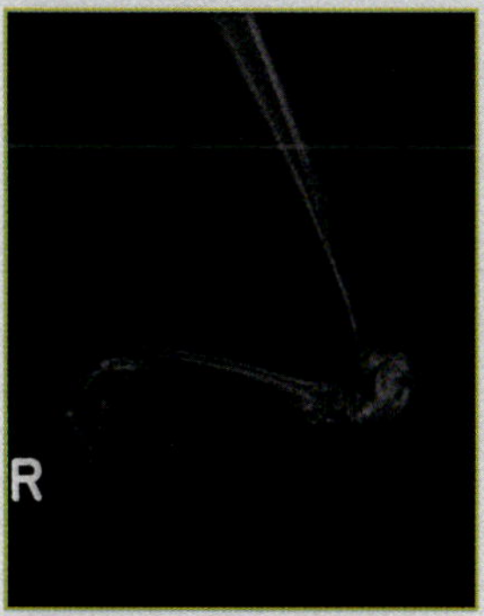

Figure 9. X-ray image of a proximal plantar intertarsal subluxation (rupture of long plantar ligament).

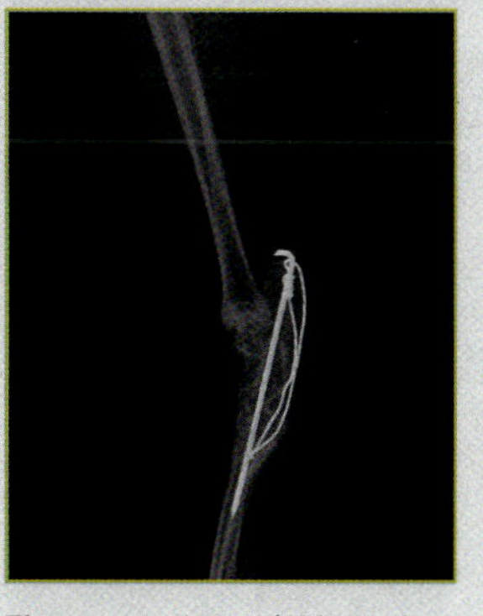

Figure 10. Lateral X-ray image of treatment using a tension band and a Steinmann pin, from the tuber calcanei through the fourth tarsal bone and third metatarsal bone.

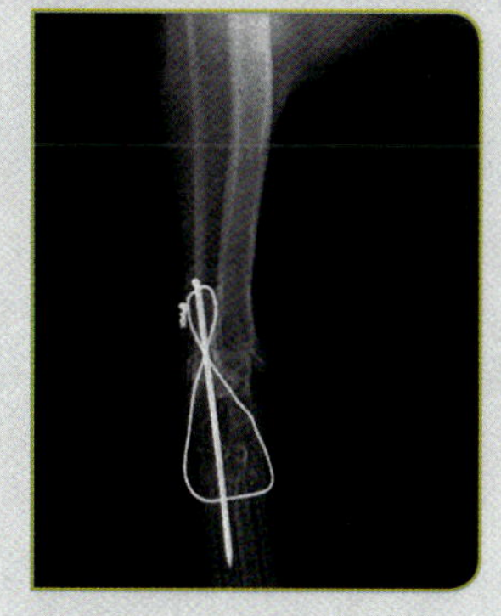

Figure 11. Dorsoplantar view of the surgery described in Figure 10.

The Steinmann pin must be fully inserted into the calcaneus to prevent irritation of the common calcaneal tendon. It is left slightly protruding on the dorsal side of the metatarsals to facilitate removal. The proximal perforation for insertion of the tension band is drilled just on the medullary cavity, cranially to the pin. The dorsal perforation is drilled on the plantar part of the fourth tarsal bone. In every other regard, plantar tarsometatarsal subluxation is treated in the same way as above.

Fractures

- With regard to **tibiotarsal fractures**, in the case of an intra-articular fracture of the talus, surgery must be performed to reduce and secure the joint with a small screw or pins, to achieve interfragmental compression.
- Another type of fracture are **fibular tarsal fractures**, which, if they are fractures of the calcaneus affecting the insertion of the gastrocnemius muscle, are treated via open reduction, with the insertion of a pin and a tension band to counterbalance muscle traction. The pin can be fully inserted into the calcaneus and remain in situ, or it may be left slightly protruding, for later removal once the fracture has healed.
- **Comminuted fractures** can be treated in a similar way; fragments can be stabilised using a cerclage, or a mini support plate can be fitted. These fractures may present concomitantly with fractures of the central tarsal bone.
- **Fractures of the talus** are uncommon but can occur. They are caused by jumps or falls. They can be fractures of the body of talus or non-articular fractures of the head or neck of talus:
    - Fractures of the **body of talus** are not always articular: this is case of those where a complete separation occurs between the two trochlear lips and the neck of talus. Articular fractures of the body of talus are serious and have a reserved prognosis. However, this does not mean that the tarsal joint must be sacrificed. The medial or lateral trochlear lip may be affected (this is difficult to observe on an X-ray), or it may be a complete fracture of the trochlear lip through the cochlea of the tibia, or an isolated fracture of a portion of one of the lips. Any fragments of cartilage must be removed, and larger osteocartilage pieces must be reduced using Kirschner wire. In some cases a malleolar osteotomy is required to expose the joint.
    - Non-articular fractures of the **head or neck of the talus** have a more positive prognosis. Minor, non-displaced fractures of the neck of the talus can be resolved successfully with external immobilisation, placing the tarsus in a neutral position. However,is it more common to find unstable or displaced fractures of the neck of the tarsus with luxation of the body and/or head of the bone. Surgical reduction and rigid fixation is the best option for full recovery of joint function. In order to reduce the fracture, the proximal intertarsal part of the joint must be flexed dorsally and the paw placed in valgus. The reduction of the fracture is held in place from the dorsal and plantar regions while a compression screw or Kirschner wire is fitted along the fracture line. Another possibility is to fit a positioning screw between the body of the talus and the calcaneus, through the tarsal canal. Fractures of the head of the talus are, in general, dorsal, often associated with fractures to the central tarsal bone. A compression screw must be fitted from the dorsomedial region.

Proximal and distal dorsal intertarsal subluxation and dorsal tarsometatarsal subluxation can generally be resolved using conservative treatment, provided that the bones of the joint can be repositioned. Where surgery is required, the joint is secured using Kirschner wire.

In general, surgical access to the tarsus is made directly, as there are no significant muscular bodies to consider. Nerves, blood vessels and tendons must be protected and retracted.

As regards, post-operative care, in the majority of cases the joint is splinted or strapped for 4 weeks, to limit forced extension and flexion, followed by a further 2 weeks of limited exercise.

03 Medial tarsal abrasion

In severe cases of abrasive injury to the medial side of the tarsus (Fig. 12), we encounter damage to the skin, soft tissue, destruction of the medial collateral ligament, tendons and joint capsule, wear and occasionally destruction of not only the malleolus but the talus, primarily affecting the trochlea, with partial or complete erosion of the medial lip. If over a quarter of the thickness of the trochlea lip has worn away, degenerative joint disease is probable.

Surgery basically consists of short and long collateral ligament plasty (Figs. 13 and 14) and temporary pinning for 4-6 weeks using external fixtures. If over 25 % of the joint surface is affected, arthrodesis should be considered.

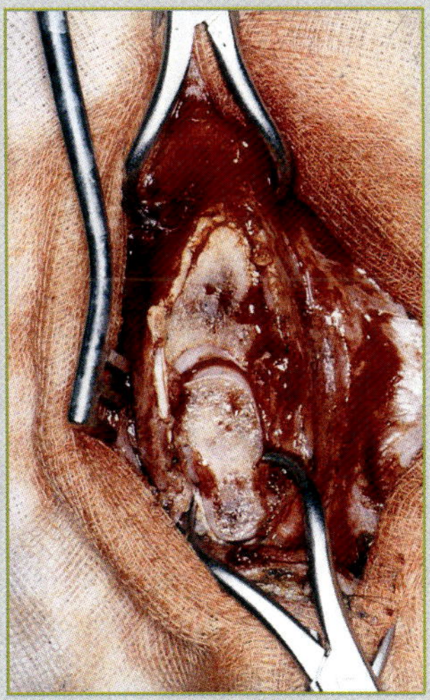

Figure 12. Damage to skin and soft tissue, destruction of medial collateral ligament, tendons and joint capsule, and erosion and complete wear to the malleolus.

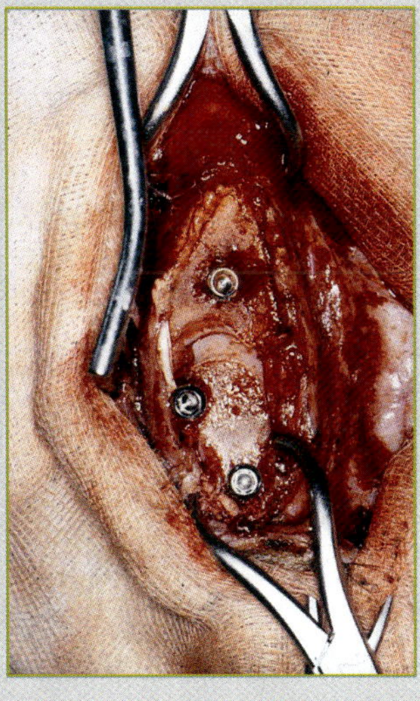

Figure 13. Surgical repair by short and long collateral ligament plasty. Self-absorbing sutures are used (therefore not visible on the X-ray).

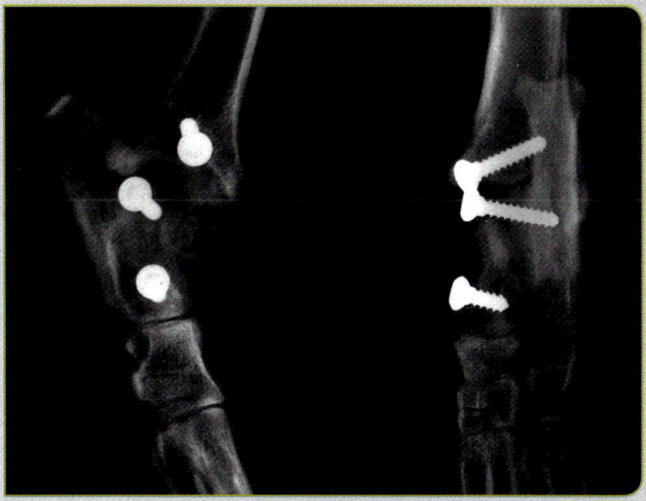

Figure 14. X-ray image of a case after 6 weeks.

04

Osteochondritis dissecans of the talus

Osteochondritis dissecans of the talus is damage to the trochlear lip. It is more common in young dogs of large breeds. Clinical signs may appear from 4 months of age. The most commonly affected breeds are: Labrador, Rottweiler, Bull Mastiff, Golden Retriever and Brazilian Mastiff. Unlike other types of osteochondrosis, females appear to be more susceptible.

Symptoms include: lameness of the pelvic limb with a short step, often together with hyperextension of the tarsal joint, and joint effusion, more common in the medial area and smaller if present on the lateral side.

The animal shows pain on flexion and extension of the joint and the range of flexion may be limited.

X-ray confirmation can be difficult. Excellent technique and oblique projections are required, such as the 15° dorsoplantar oblique angle, to avoid overlapping of the calcaneus with the trochlear lips.

Appropriate projections for the X-ray study of the medial or lateral trochlear lip are shown in Table 1.

Table 1. Radiological projections for study of the trochlea.

Study of the medial trochlear lip:
- Dorsoplantar.
- Lateromedial.
- Lateromedial in flexion, used for the study of the proximal end of the trochlear lips.
- Dorsolateral-planteromedial oblique (Figs. 15 and 16).

Study of the lateral trochlear lip:
- Lateromedial.
- Lateromedial in flexion.
- 30°/45° Dorsolateral-planteromedial oblique.
- Dorsoplantar in flexion, with the animal in lateral recumbency, taking images at different angles of flexion.

15
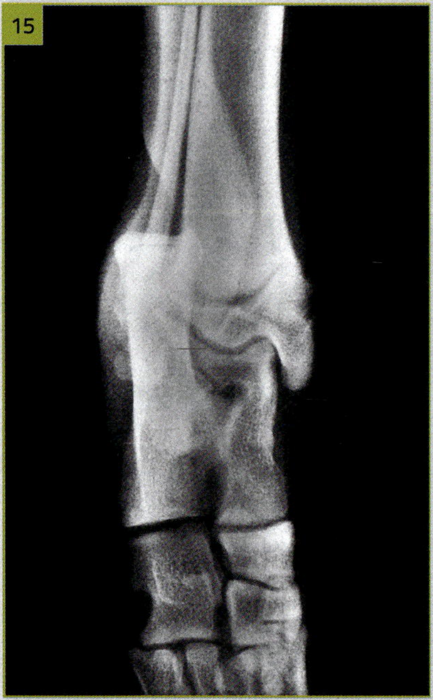

16
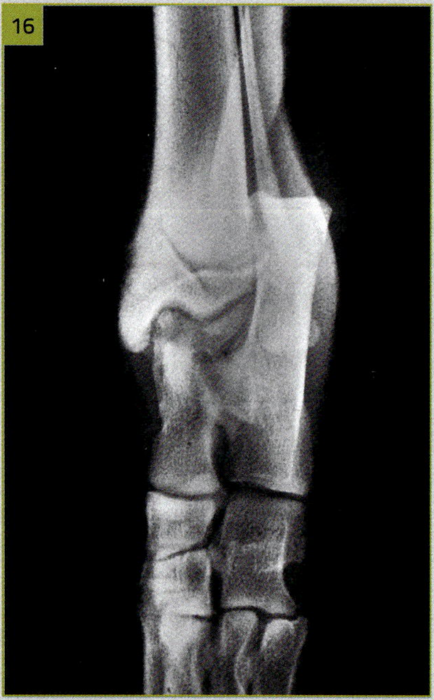

Figure 15. X-ray image using a dorsolateral-planteromedial oblique for the study of the medial trochlear lip of the talus.

Figure 16. Contralateral X-ray image using an oblique dorsolateral-planteromedial projection for the study of the medial trochlear lip of the talus.

Radiologically identifiable damage includes a flattened trochlear lip and/or an enlarged joint space (Fig. 17).

Statistically, damage is more common on the medial lip, occurring in 75 % of cases. Statistic also show that damage to the lateral lip is more common in the Rottweiler.

Damage may appear at any point along the lip, but more in the caudal or cranial plantar part. Sometimes damage may appear on both lips.

In 44 % of cases damage is bilateral, although it is unusual for the dog to suffer concurrent osteochondritis dissecans in other joints.

Despite controversy about the efficacy of surgery, most surgeons opt to remove the piece of cartilage or osteochondral fragment.

The least traumatic surgical approaches are dorsomedial, plantar medial, dorsolateral and plantar lateral. For damage to the medial lip, surgery consists of approaching the joint from the caudal area without osteotomy of the malleoleus or tenotomy, with the joint in maximum flexion. The trochlea is palpated with the finger, and the incision is made in the capsule, protecting the caudal tibial muscle tendon and the deep digital flexor muscle tendon, and the entire caudal and dorsal compartment is examined. If necessary, the most cranial part can be visualised, another arthrotomy is performed between the medial collateral ligament and the cranial tibial muscle tendon. During the procedure, care must be taken not to damage the saphenous nerve, the dorsal and caudal branches of the saphenous artery and vein and the cranial tibial artery and vein. Debridement and curettage is performed on the damaged tissue. It has never been possible to verify or document the efficacy of a perforation in the subchondral bone in dogs.

No external immobilisation is required during the postoperative period. An oedema appears, which will be reabsorbed within two weeks. Lameness should disappear within around 20 days.

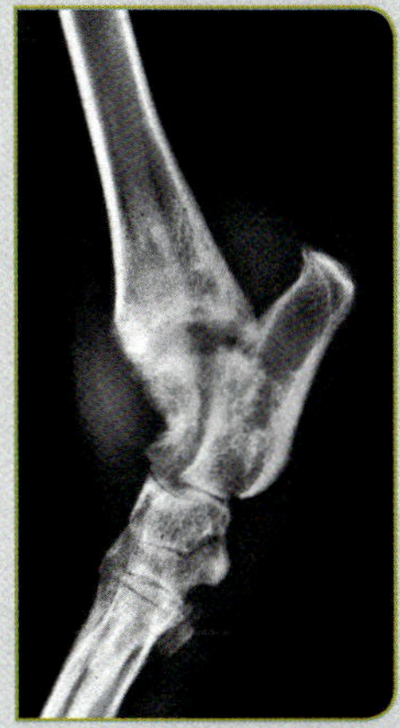

Figure 17. Radiologically identifiable damage includes a flattened trochlear lip and/or an enlarged joint space.

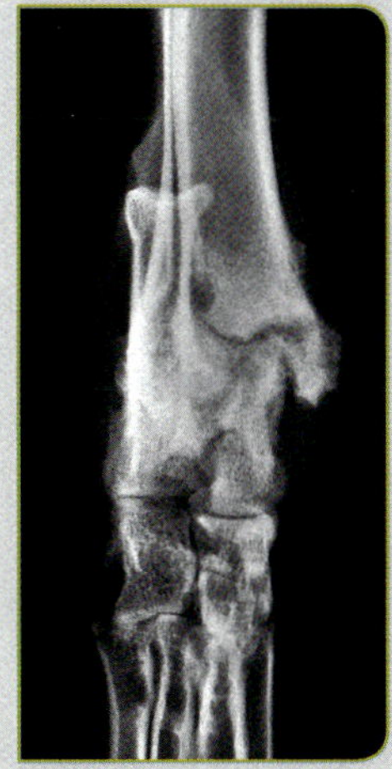

Figure 18. In severe cases of osteoarthritis, such as the one shown here, arthrodesis should be considered.

Today, transmalleolar access via an osteotomy of the malleolus is no longer the procedure of choice, and is only required on rare occasions. Furthermore, it is difficult to perform malleolar osteotomy correctly as it must be deep enough to include the malleolus and the medial collateral ligament, but not deep enough to affect the weight-bearing part of the joint surface.

Another approach is via fibular osteotomy, which may indicated in the case of distal damage to the lateral lip.

Post-surgical X-ray images often show degenerative arthropathy caused by joint instability of incongruity (Fig. 18). A slight, but noticeable lameness may occasionally persist.

It is important to note that, in some cases during the exploratory arthrotomy damage fragments are not visible, and only changes in the colour of the damages cartilage are observed.

Arthrodesis and pan-arthrodesis

Tarsal arthrodesis is indicated in cases of severe joint abrasion, painful arthropathy, irreparable or long-term fractures, irreparable injuries of the common calcaneus tendon, and damage to the sciatic nerve. If the damage to the talus or its points of articulation is so severe that effective reconstruction is not possible, arthrodesis may be indicated.

This is the great challenge faced by orthopaedic veterinary surgeons. While it is more easily performed in cats, this procedure is not always advisable in this species. Cats recover very poorly from arthrodesis of the tarsal (and stifle) joints, meaning that an X-ray of an irreparable yet functional tarsus may be preferable to a perfectly executed yet non-functional arthrodesis.

The basic conditions for successful arthrodesis are:

1. Complete removal of the joint cartilage.
2. Transplant of sufficient autogenous spongy tissue.
3. Firm stabilisation of the joints to be fused.

A number of techniques have been established to stabilise the joints; for example: traction screws, dorsal (Figs. 19-22), medial or lateral plates and external pins. The purpose of all these techniques is to immobilise the talocrural joint, which is the most mobile.

A review of available literature shows that the tarsal joint is not easily immobilised. The success rate is somewhere between 50-65 %. Failure is generally due to a high rate of complications, such as: loosening or breakage of implants, osteomyelitis, failure of bone consolidation and arthropathy in the intertarsal or tarsometatarsal joints. Insufficient stabilisation is the most common source of complications, as instability delays immobilisation and places excess load on the implants, eventually resulting in loosening or breakage. The cause of insufficient stability may be poorly chosen or incorrectly fitted implants. For this reason it is advisable to protect them using a case or other similar method.

An analysis of the complications of arthrodesis of the tarsus shows that in the majority of cases these are caused by insufficient stabilisation of the calcaneus. Despite the greatest movement taking place in the talocrural joint, there is also a certain level of movement between the calcaneus and the talus. This is due to the tension of the calcaneal tendon over the calcaneus.

Our experience leads us to recommend the process shown in Table 2.

Table 2. Recommendations for performing arthrodesis.

1. If arthrodesis of the talocrural joint is required, it is advisable to perform a pan-arthrodesis.
2. The best stabilisation method is the use of a dorsal plate.
3. The size of the plate used is determined by the diameter of screw that can be inserted into the metatarsal.
4. The length of the plate must allow at least 3 screws to be used on the tibia and a further 3 on the third metatarsal.
5. A minimum of 2 screws must be fitted, one on the talus and another on the calcaneus, in the middle section of the plate. This blocks the joint and reduces strain on the plate.
6. To achieve full, effective and painless immobilisation, i.e. free of lameness, rigid fixing of the calcaneus is required.

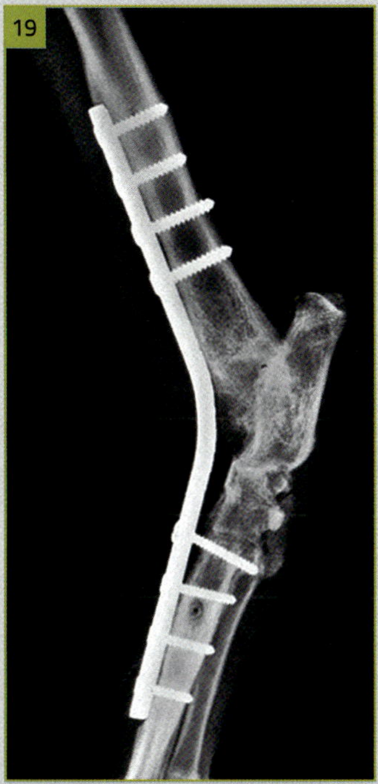

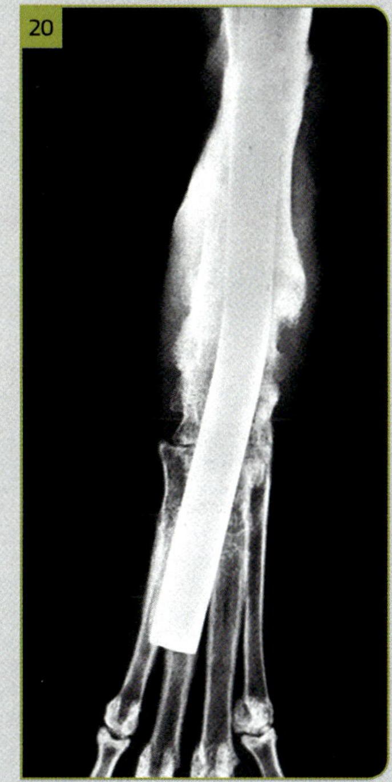

Figure 19. Lateral X-ray image of a pan-arthrodesis using a dorsal plate, 6 months after surgery.

Figure 20. Dorsoplantar X-ray image of a pan-arthrodesis using a dorsal plate, 6 months after surgery.

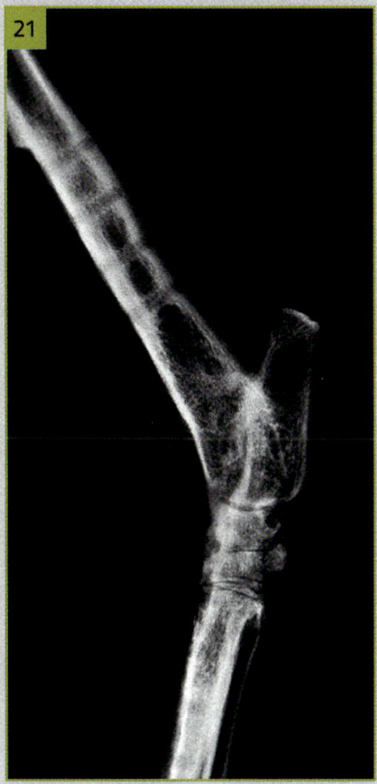

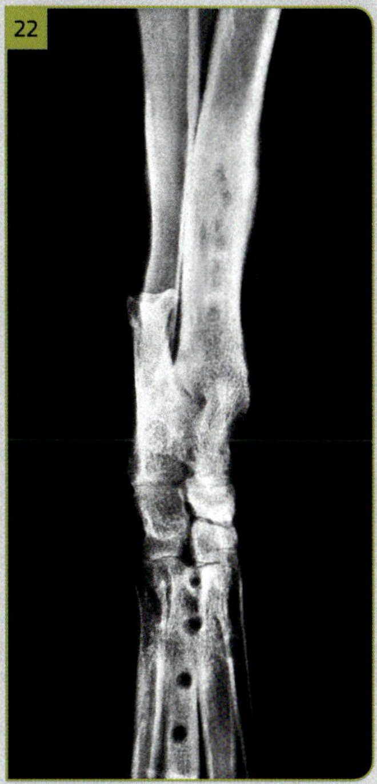

Figure 21. Lateral X-ray image of a pan-arthrodesis after removal of the implant.

Figure 22. Dorsal X-ray image of a pan-arthrodesis after removal of the implant.

Diagnostic imaging techniques

The following are pairs of images comparing transparent plastinated sections of real structures compared with images obtained using CAT and MRI.

Transparent plastinated sections + CAT

Carpal joint

SAGITTAL SECTION OF THE CARPAL JOINT

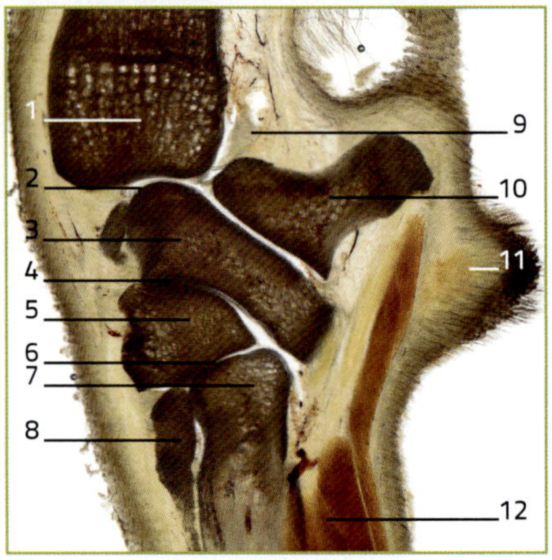

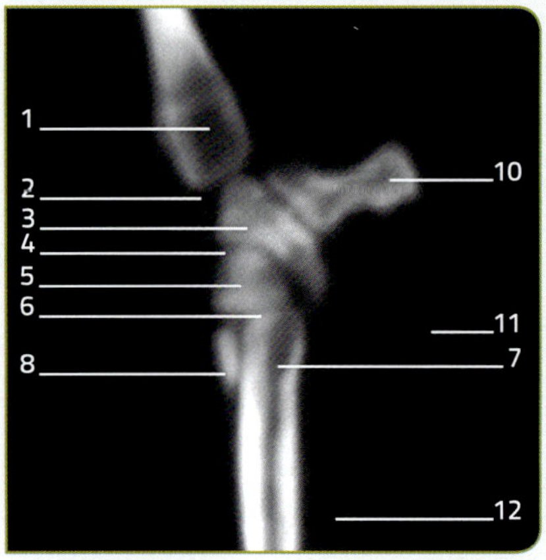

1	Trochlea of the radius
2	Antebrachiocarpal joint
3	Carpoulnar bone
4	Intercarpal joint
5	Fourth carpal bone
6	Carpometacarpal joint
7	Fifth metacarpal bone
8	Fourth metacarpal bone
9	Joint capsule
10	Accessory bone
11	Carpal torus
12	Interosseous muscle

HORIZONTAL OR DORSAL SECTION OF THE CARPAL JOINT

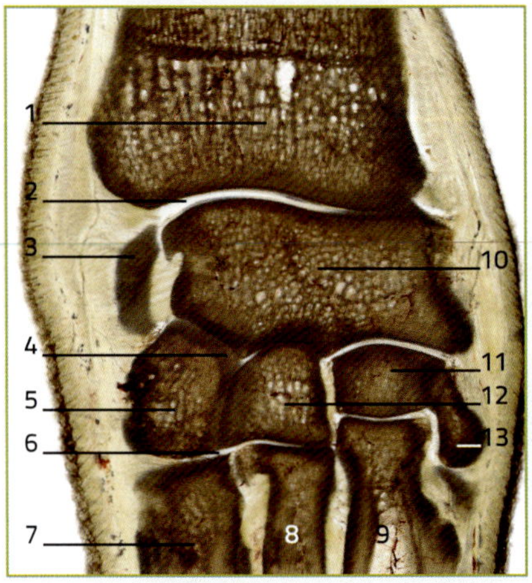

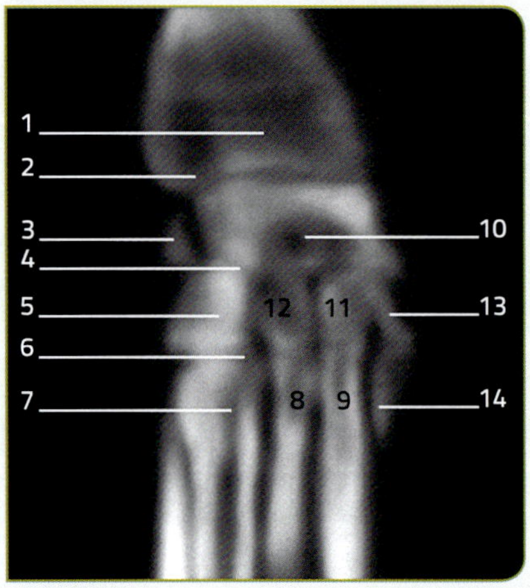

1	Trochlea of the radius
2	Antebrachiocarpal joint
3	Carpoulnar bone
4	Intercarpal joint
5	Fourth carpal bone
6	Carpometacarpal joint
7	Fourth metacarpal bone
8	Third metacarpal bone
9	Second metacarpal bone
10	Intermediate radial bone
11	Second carpal bone
12	Third carpal bone
13	First carpal bone
14	First metacarpal bone

Tarsal joint

SAGITTAL SECTION OF THE TARSUS IN SEMI-FLEXION

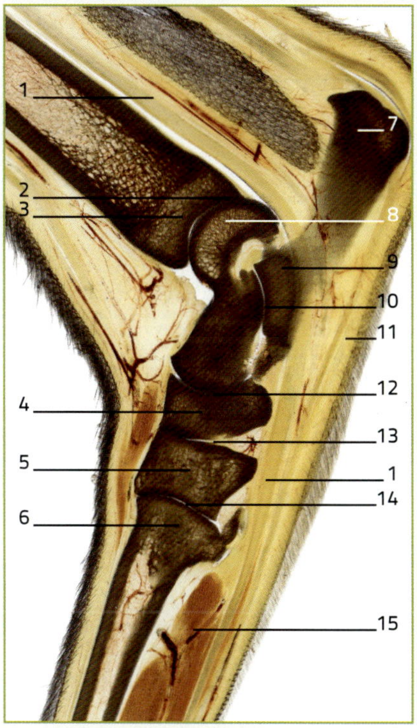

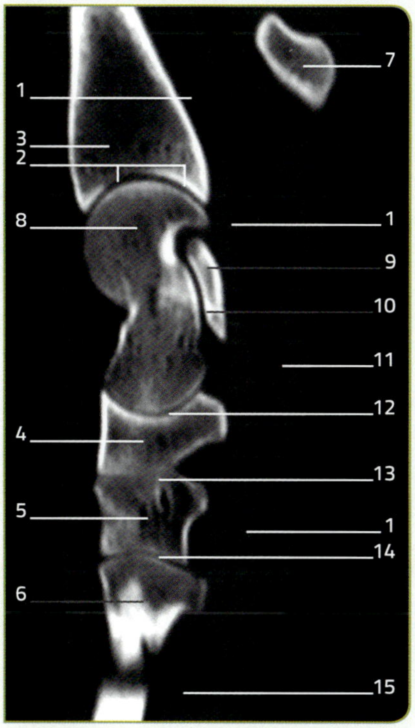

1	Lateral digital flexor muscle tendon
2	Talocrural joint
3	Tibial cochlea
4	Central tarsal bone
5	Third tarsal bone
6	Second metatarsal bone
7	Tuber calcanei
8	Trochlea of the talus
9	Sustentaculum tali
10	Talocalcaneal joint
11	Superficial digital flexor muscle tendon
12	Proximal intertarsal joint
13	Distal intertarsal joint
14	Tarsometatarsal joint
15	Interosseous muscles

Transparent plastinated sections + MRI

Carpal joint

SAGITTAL SECTION OF THE CARPAL JOINT

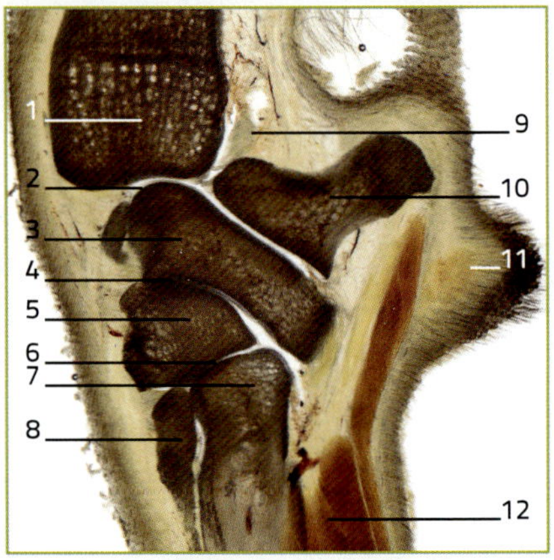

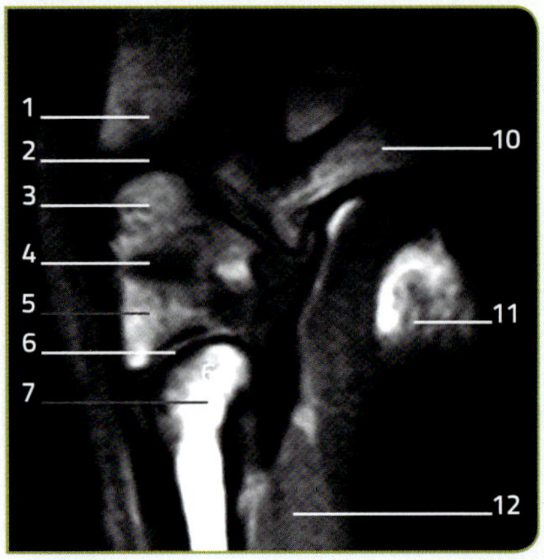

1	Trochlea of the radius
2	Antebrachiocarpal joint
3	Carpoulnar bone
4	Intercarpal joint
5	Fourth carpal bone
6	Carpometacarpal joint
7	Fifth metacarpal bone
8	Fourth metacarpal bone
9	Joint capsule
10	Accessory bone
11	Carpal torus
12	Interosseous muscle

HORIZONTAL OR DORSAL SECTION OF THE CARPAL JOINT

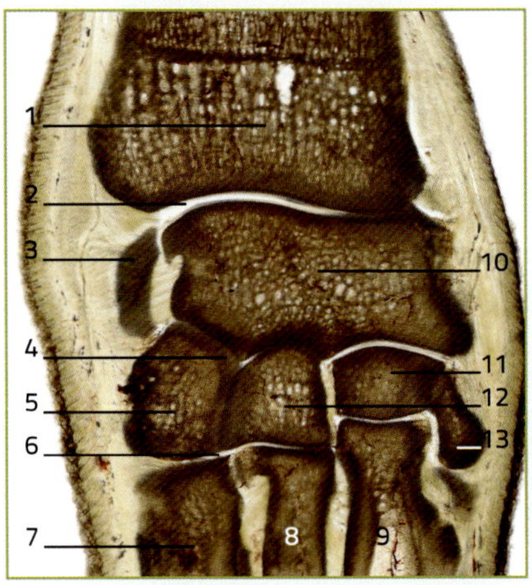

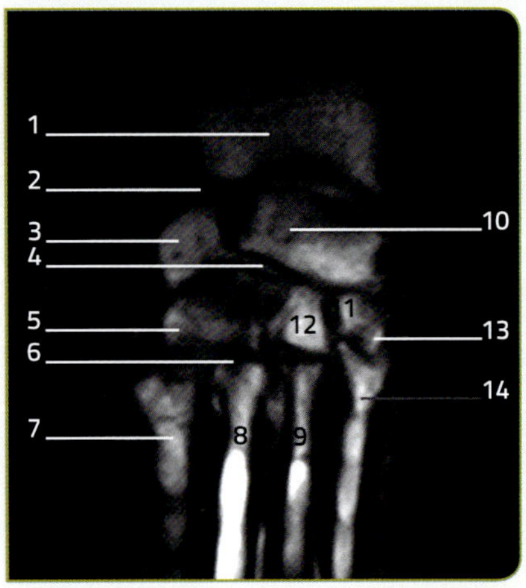

1	Trochlea of the radius
2	Antebrachiocarpal joint
3	Carpoulnar bone
4	Intercarpal joint
5	Fourth carpal bone
6	Carpometacarpal joint
7	Fourth metacarpal bone
8	Third metacarpal bone
9	Second metacarpal bone
10	Intermediate radial bone
11	Second carpal bone
12	Third carpal bone
13	First carpal bone
14	First metacarpal bone

Tarsal joint

SAGITTAL SECTION OF THE TARSUS IN SEMI-FLEXION

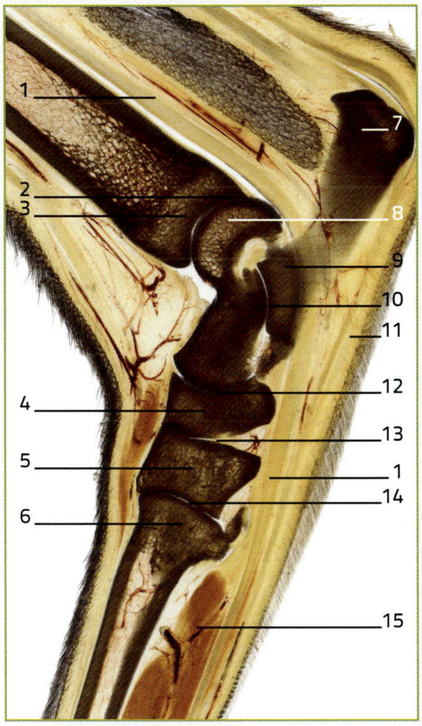

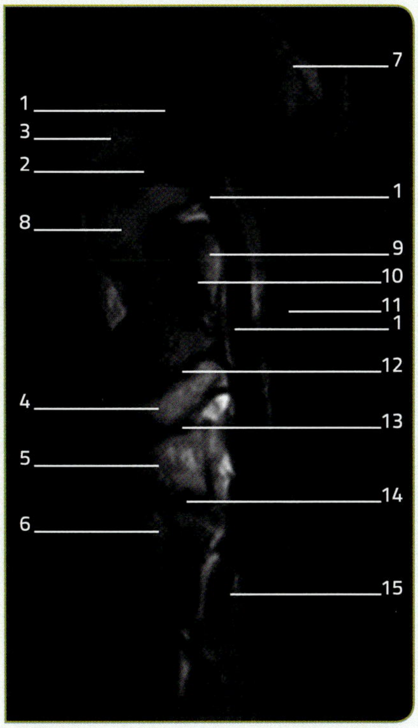

1	Lateral digital flexor muscle tendon
2	Talocrural joint
3	Tibial cochlea
4	Central tarsal bone
5	Third tarsal bone
6	Second metatarsal bone
7	Tuber calcanei
8	Trochlea of the talus
9	Sustentaculum tali
10	Talocalcaneal joint
11	Superficial digital flexor muscle tendon
12	Proximal intertarsal joint
13	Distal intertarsal joint
14	Tarsometatarsal joint
15	Interosseous muscles

SURGICAL APPROACHES

Carpal joint

Dorsal approach to the carpal joint

1 The skin incision runs along the dorsal side of the carpal joint, from the medial edge of the forearm to the lateral edge of the fifth metacarpal bone (dotted line). Right forelimb.

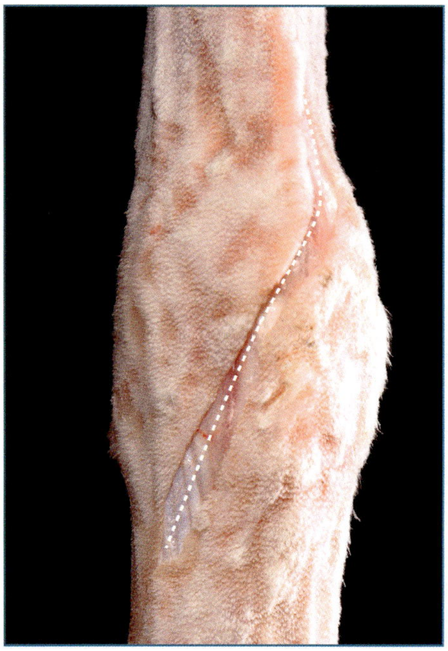

2 Subcutaneously, the tendons of the common digital extensor muscle, the lateral digital extensor muscle and the radial carpal extensor muscle are located. The carpal fascia and the blood vessels of the dorsal side of the joint should be displaced medially (dotted line).
Warning: the course of the accessory cephalic vein must be avoided.

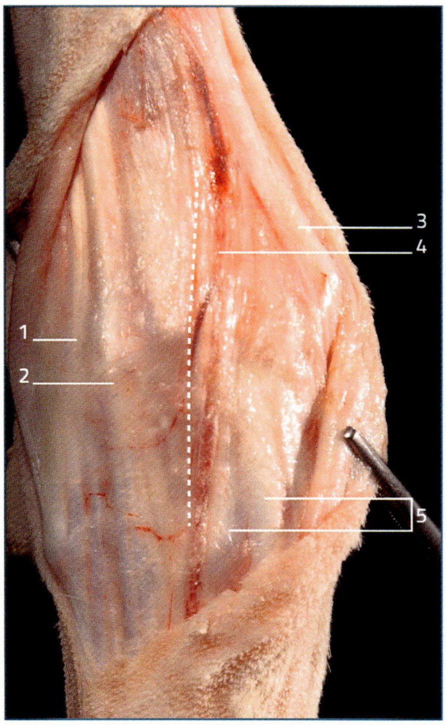

1 Lateral digital extensor muscle tendon
2 Common digital extensor muscle tendon
3 Long abductor muscle tendon of the first toe
4 Accessory cephalic vein
5 Carpal radial extensor muscle tendon

3 After medial displacement of the blood vessels, the joint capsule is located and incised between the extensor carpi radialis tendon and the common digital extensor tendon (dotted line).

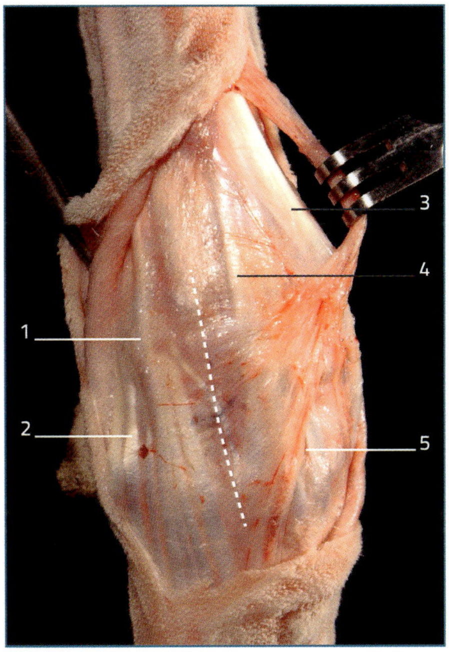

1 Common digital extensor muscle tendon
2 Lateral digital extensor muscle tendon
3 Long abductor muscle tendon of the first toe
4 Extensor carpi radialis muscle tendon
5 Accessory cephalic vein

4 After sectioning the capsule and exerting slight semi-flexion on the antebrachiocarpal joint, the joint surface of the carpal bones can be exposed.

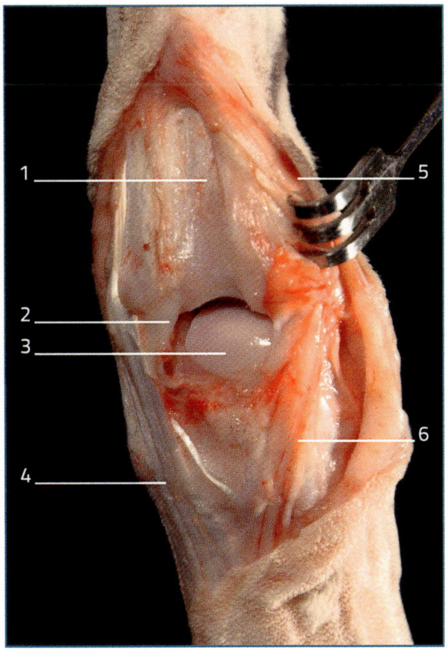

1 Radius
2 Joint capsule
3 Proximal joint surface of the intermediate radial bone
4 Common digital extensor muscle tendon
5 Long abductor muscle tendon of the the first toe
6 Accessory cephalic vein

Palmar medial approach to the carpal joint

1 The skin incision runs along the medial edge of the carpal joint, from the distal end of the radius to the palmar surface of the metacarpals (dotted line). The first toe has been amputated in the animal dissected here. Palmar medial view of the right paw.

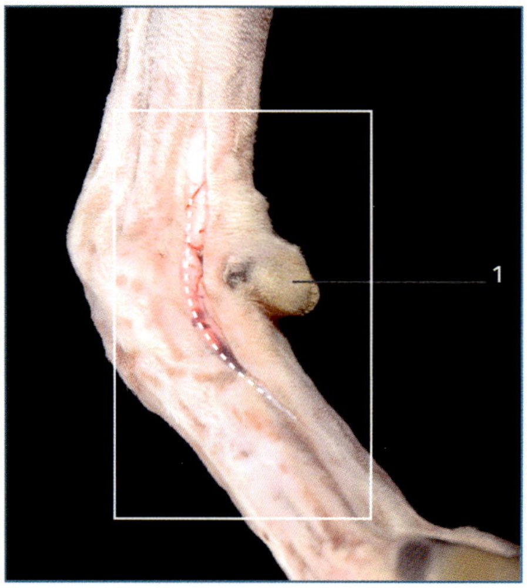

1 Carpal torus (carpal pad)

2 Subcutaneously, the tendons of the superficial digital flexor muscle and the radial carpal flexor muscle are located. The flexor retinaculum and the cephalic vein must be sectioned and ligated respectively (dotted line) in order to access the palmar surface of the carpal joint.
Warning: take care to avoid damage to the cephalic vein.

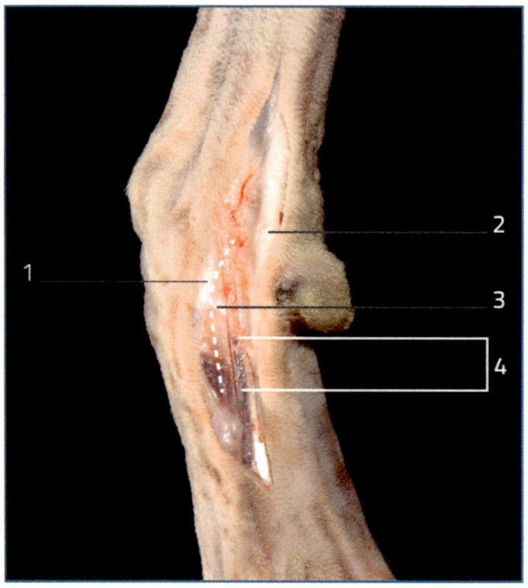

1 Carpal radial flexor muscle tendon
2 Superficial digital flexor muscle tendon
3 Flexor retinaculum
4 Cephalic vein

3 Sectioning of the flexor retinaculum exposes the carpal canal, the deep digital flexor muscle tendon and the course of the median artery and nerve. The deep digital flexor tendon for the first toe has been sectioned to allow greater exposure of the carpal joint.

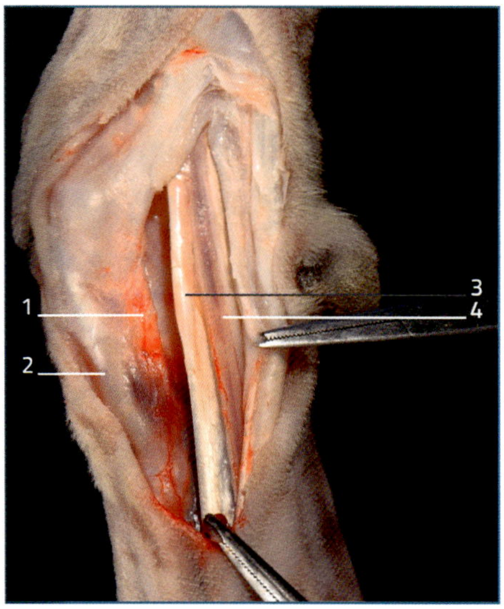

1 Joint capsule
2 First metacarpal
3 Deep digital flexor muscle tendon
4 Median artery and nerve

4 The superficial and deep digital flexor tendons and the median nerve and vascular supply are displaced laterally to expose the palmar surface of the carpal joint. The joint capsule and palmar carpal ligaments are incised after identifying the interosseous spaces (dotted line).

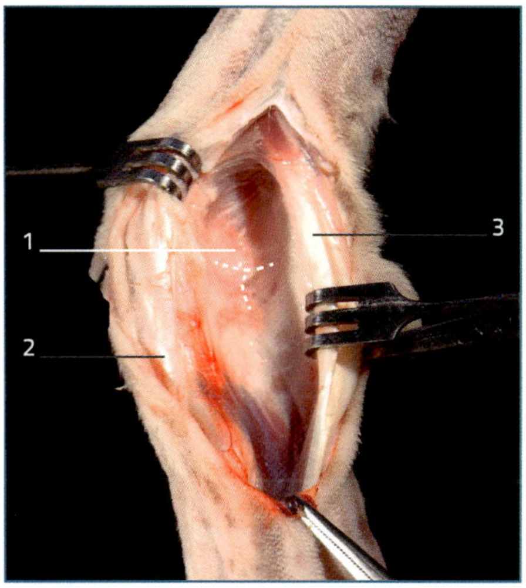

1 Joint capsule
2 First metacarpal
3 Deep digital flexor muscle tendon

5 Sectioning the joint capsule allows a palmar approach to the different bones of the carpal joint.
Warning: care must be taken during incision of the joint capsule to avoid the deep palmar vessels and the palmar metacarpal arteries (see following image).

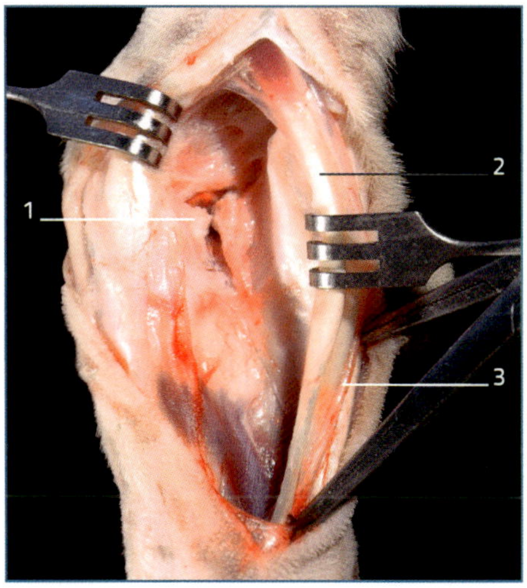

1 Joint capsule
2 Deep digital flexor muscle tendon
3 Median artery and nerve

6 Dissection of the main arteries of the palmar side of the manus. The superficial and deep digital flexor muscle tendons have been removed, and the medial artery and common palmar digital arteries have been left intact and displaced medially.

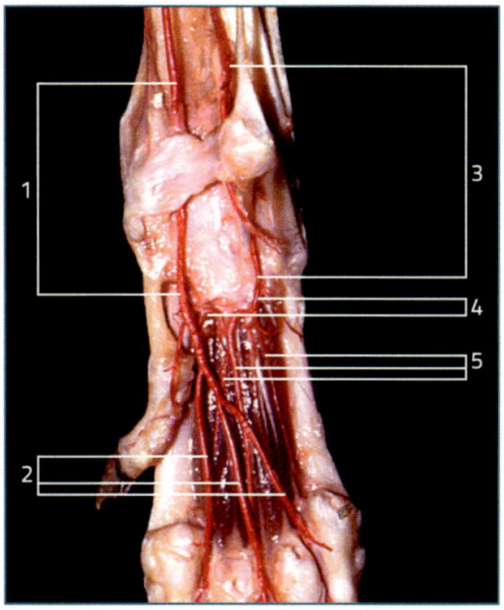

1 Median artery
2 Common palmar digital arteries
3 Caudal interosseous artery
4 Deep palmar vessels
5 Palmar metacarpal arteries

Tarsal joint

Approach to the lateral malleolus and the talocrural joint

1 The skin incision runs along the lateral malleolus of the fibula and extends to the distal end of the tarsus. Right hind limb.

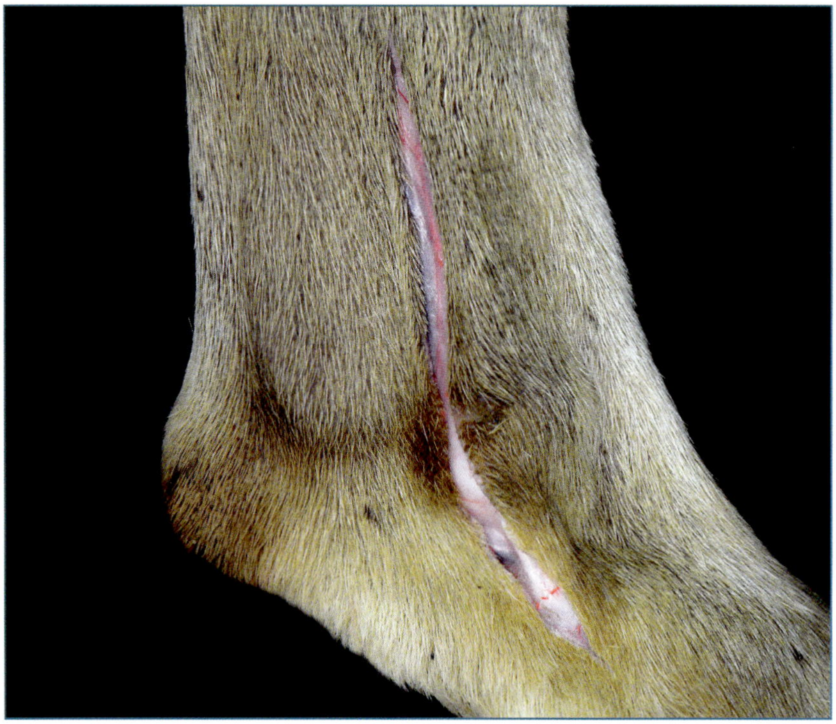

2 The tendons of the long fibular muscle, lateral digital extensor muscle and short fibular muscle are identified on their course through the malleolar sulci. The retinaculum must be sectioned to expose the lateral malleolus.

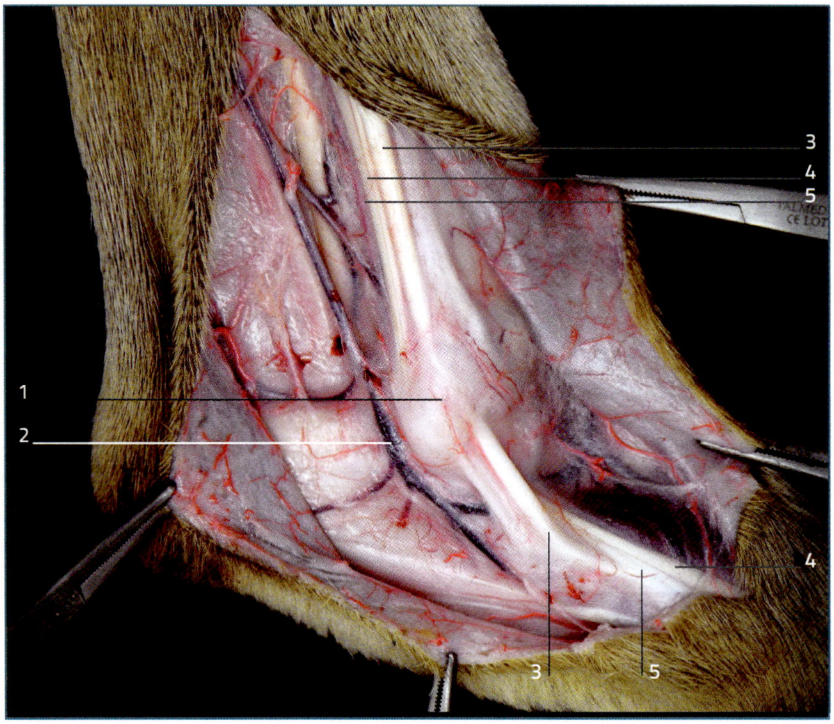

1 Retinaculum of the fibular muscles
2 Caudal branch of the lateral saphenous vein
3 Long fibular muscle tendon
4 Lateral digital extensor muscle tendon
5 Short fibular muscle tendon

3 The lateral malleolus is exposed by sectioning the retinaculum of the fibular muscles. To access the talocrural joint, the joint capsule must be incised between the long digital extensor and long fibular tendons, running along the trochlea of the talus.

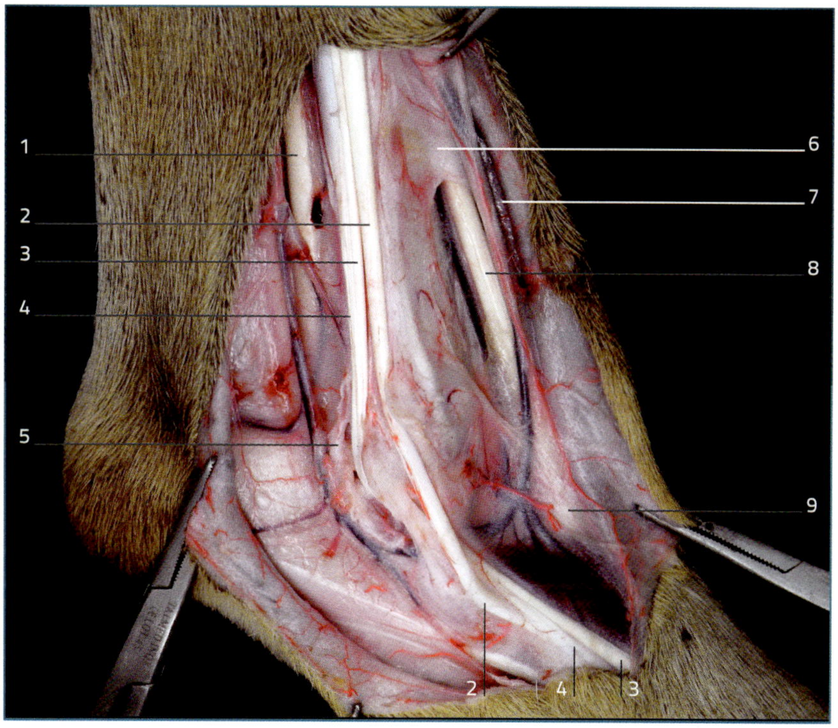

1 Lateral digital flexor muscle tendon
2 Long fibular muscle tendon
3 Lateral digital extensor muscle tendon
4 Short fibular muscle tendon
5 Retinaculum of the fibular muscles
6 Crural extensor retinaculum
7 Lateral saphenous vein
8 Long digital extensor muscle tendon
9 Tarsal extensor retinaculum

4 After sectioning of the joint capsule the trochlea of the talus is exposed. Warning: the course of the lateral saphenous vein must be avoided.

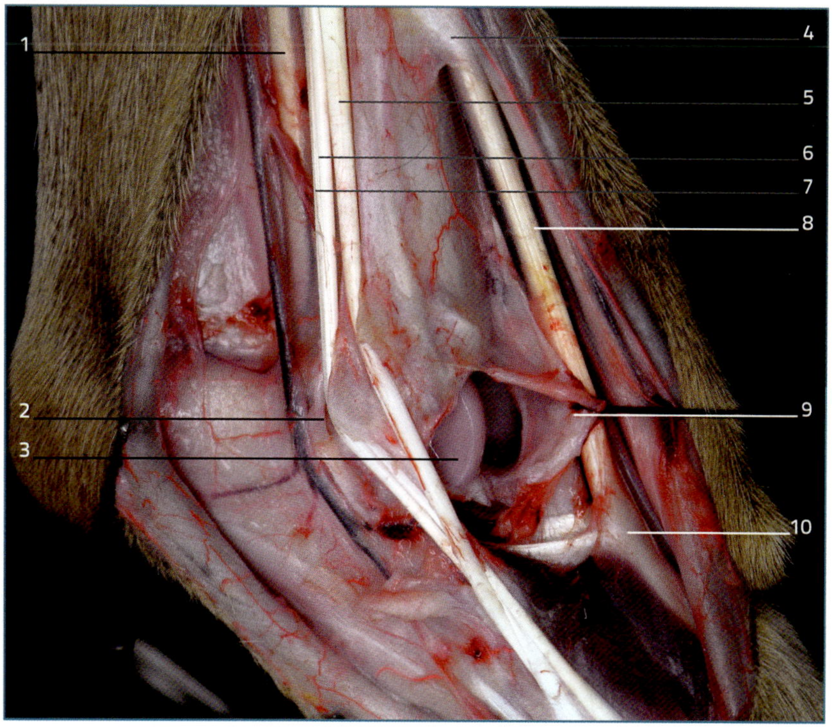

1 Lateral digital flexor muscle tendon
2 Lateral malleolar sulcus
3 Lateral lip of trochlea of the talus
4 Crural extensor retinaculum
5 Long fibular muscle tendon
6 Lateral digital extensor muscle tendon
7 Short fibular muscle tendon
8 Long digital extensor muscle tendon
9 Joint capsule
10 Tarsal extensor retinaculum

Approach to the medial malleolus and the talocrural joint

1 The skin incision runs along the medial malleolus and the base of the second metatarsal. Right hind limb.

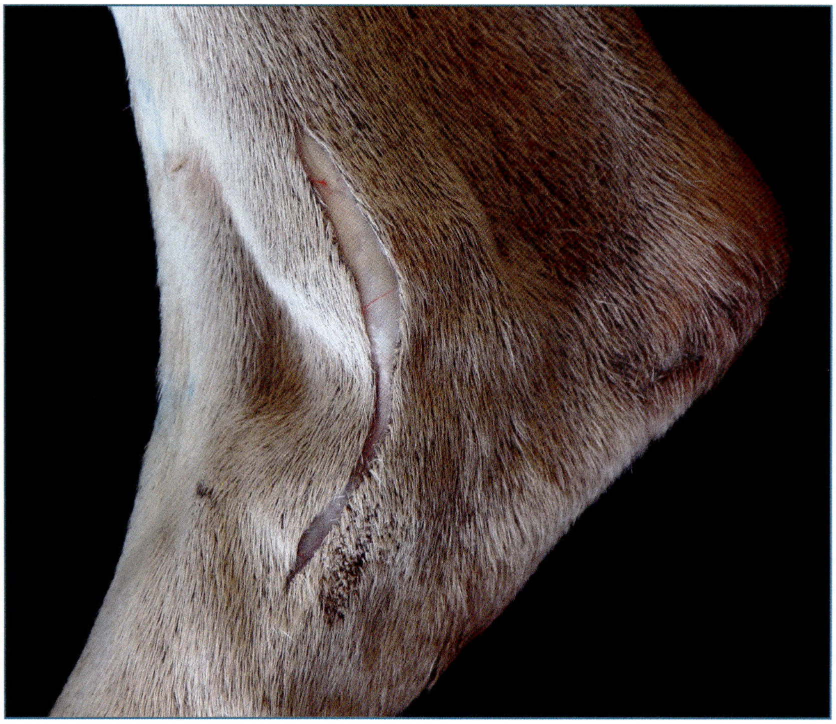

2 Subcutaneously, the medial collateral ligament and the cranial tibial muscle tendon are identified; the joint capsule is sectioned between the two. The medial malleolus is covered by the collateral ligament.

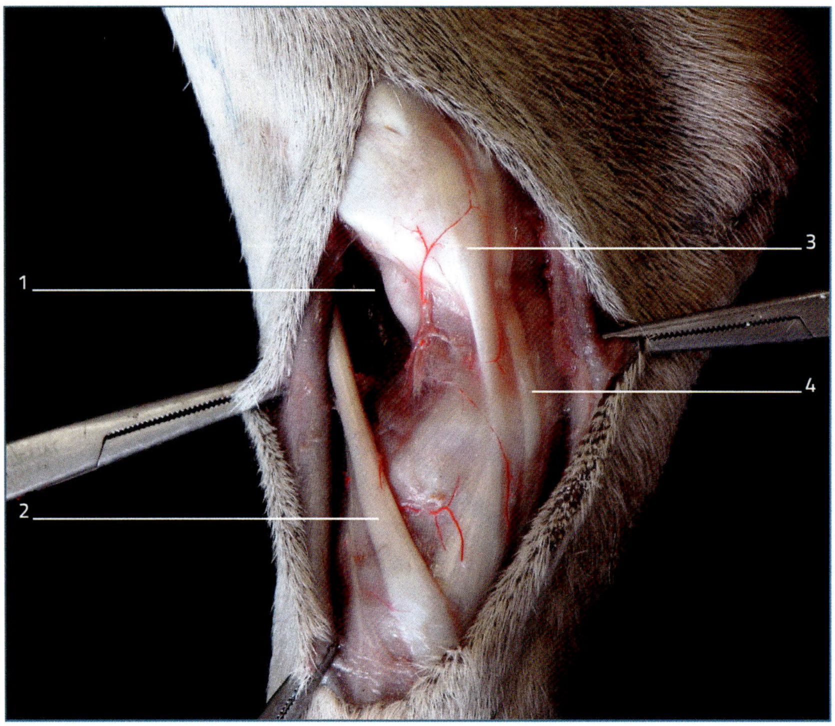

1 Joint capsule
2 Cranial tibial muscle tendon
3 Medial collateral ligament
4 Medial digital flexor muscle tendon

3 On sectioning the joint capsule the medial lip of the trochlea of the talus bone is identified.

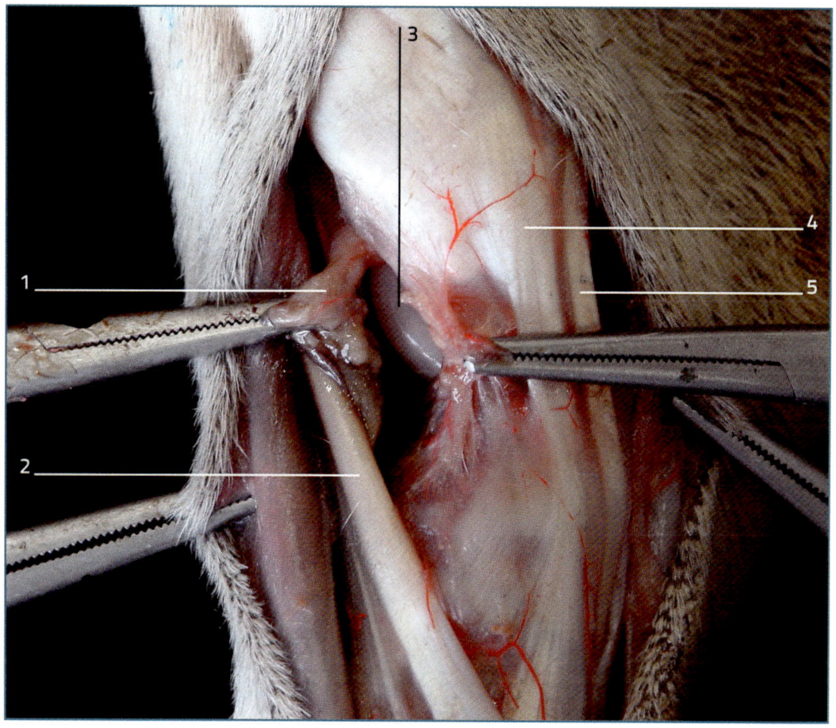

1 Joint capsule
2 Cranial tibial muscle tendon
3 Medial lip of trochlea of the talus
4 Medial collateral ligament
5 Medial digital flexor muscle tendon

4 This image shows the position of the medial collateral ligament in relation to the tendons of the caudal tibial and medial digital flexor muscles, which must be avoided if this approach is to be used for a medial malleolar osteotomy.

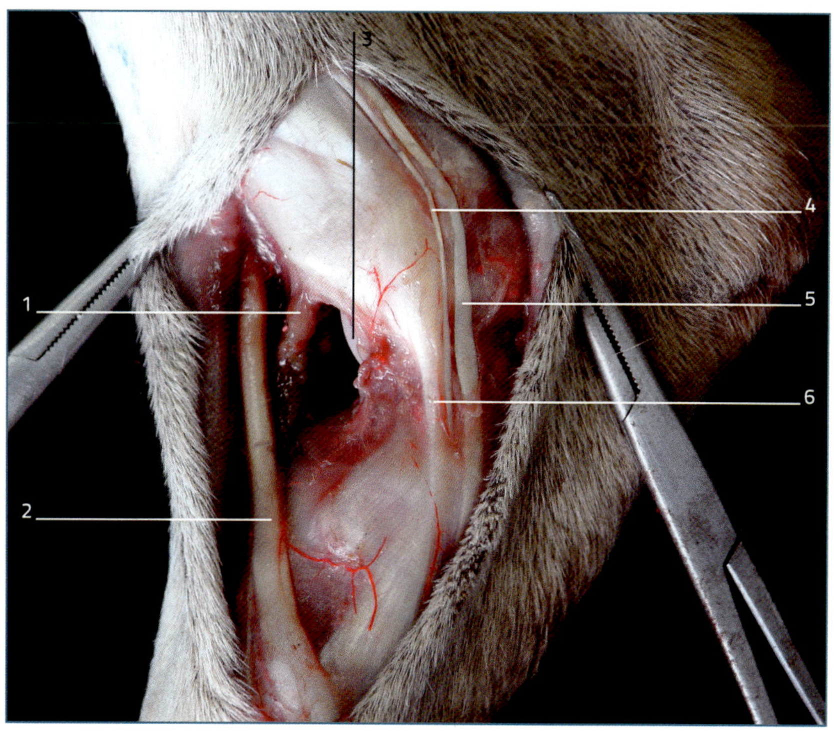

1 Joint capsule
2 Cranial tibial muscle tendon
3 Medial lip of trochlea of the talus
4 Caudal tibial muscle tendon
5 Medial digital flexor muscle tendon
6 Medial collateral ligament

Approach to the talocrural joint via osteotomy of the medial malleolus

1 A medial approach to the talocrural joint is used. The medial collateral ligament is isolated, with caudal displacement of the caudal tibial and medial digital flexor tendons. The medial malleolar osteotomy is performed close to the point of attachment of the medial collateral ligament.

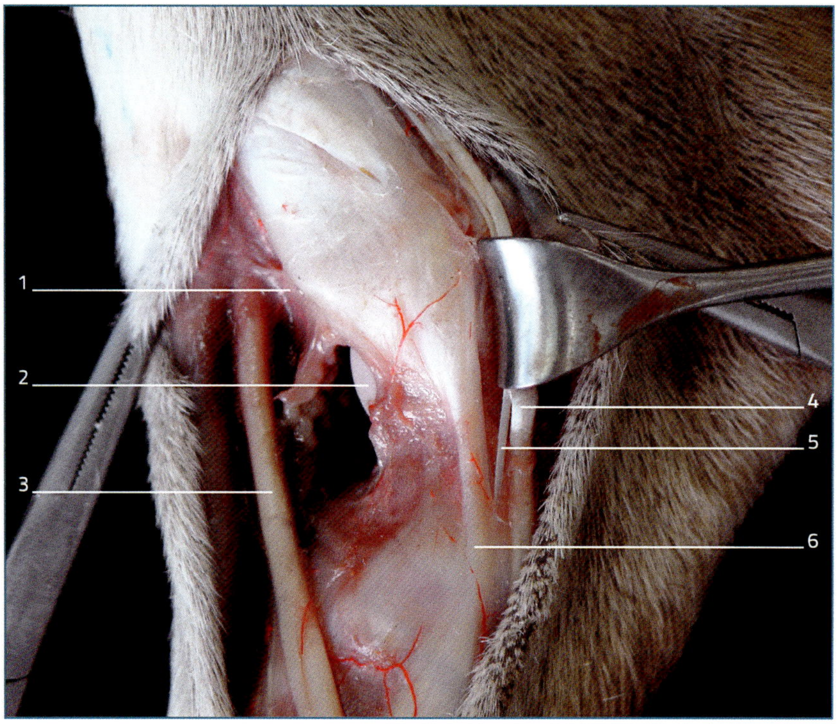

1 Joint capsule
2 Medial lip of trochlea of the talus
3 Cranial tibial muscle tendon
4 Medial digital flexor muscle tendon
5 Caudal tibial muscle tendon
6 Medial collateral ligament

2 After the osteotomy, the medial malleolus is displaced to expose the entire trochlea of the talus.

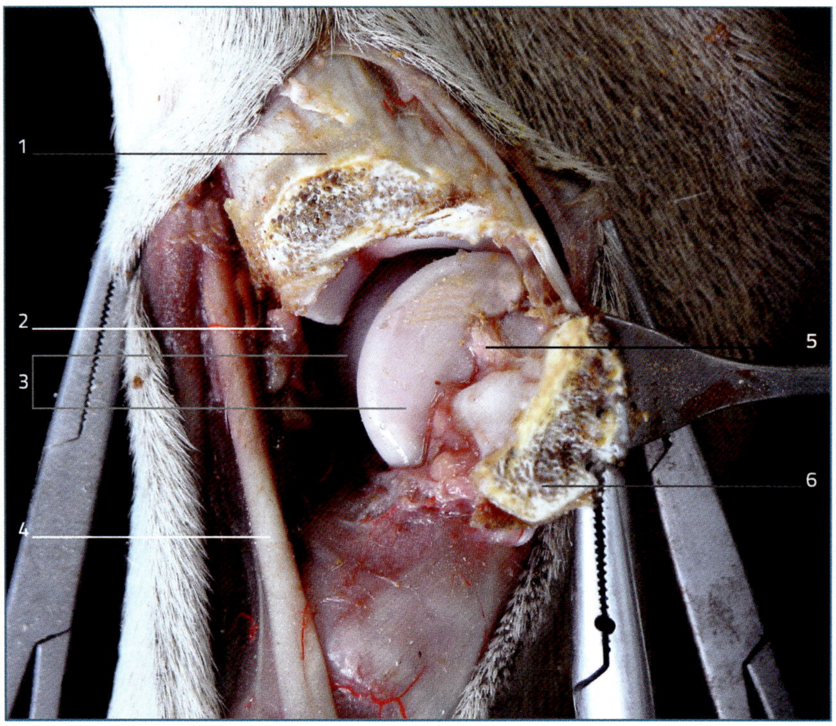

1 Tibia
2 Joint capsule
3 Medial and lateral lips of trochlea of the talus
4 Cranial tibial muscle tendon
5 Collateral ligament
6 Medial malleolus

3 Enlargement of the previous image. Note the joint cartilage covering the trochlea of the talus, and part of the tarsal joint surface of the tibia.

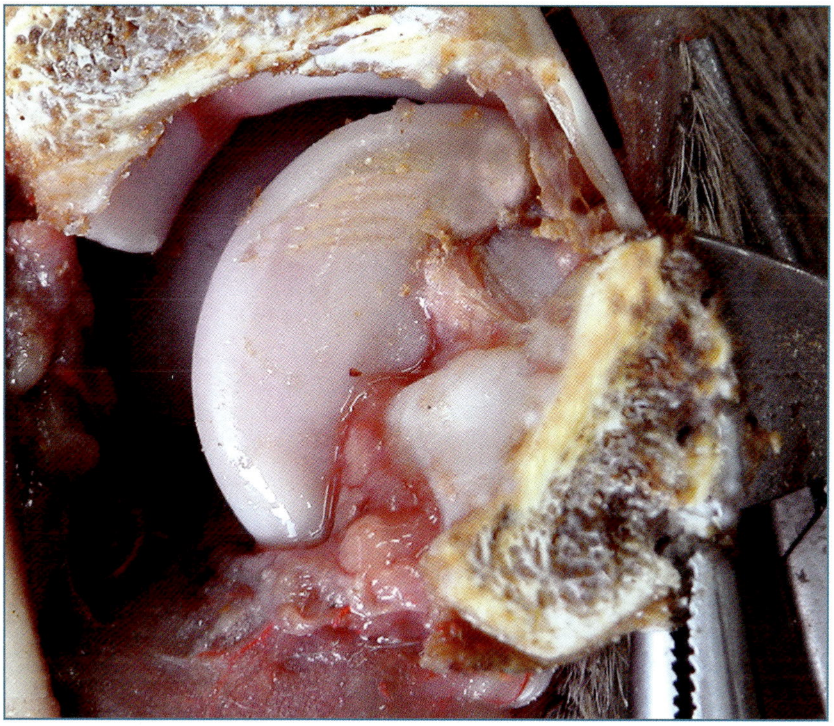

4 It can be seen how, on internal rotation of the tarsus, both lips of the trochlea of the talus can be examined.

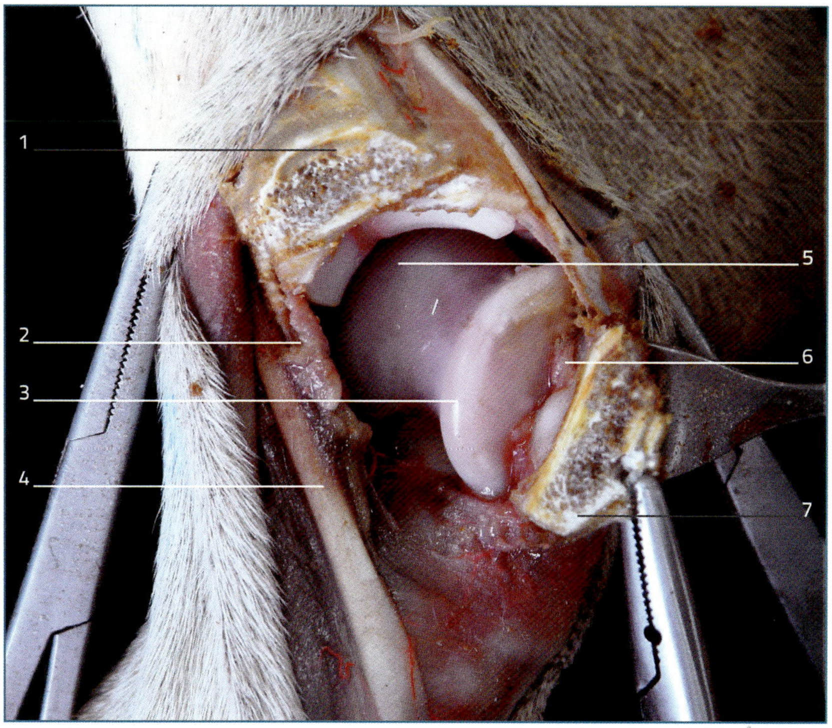

1 Tibia
2 Joint capsule
3 Medial lip of trochlea of the talus
4 Cranial tibial muscle tendon
5 Lateral lip of trochlea of the talus
6 Collateral ligament
7 Medial malleolus

Approach to the calcaneus

1 The skin incision is made over the lateral malleolus, in the direction of the plantar area. The tuber calcanei is exposed by retracting the skin medially. Right hind limb.

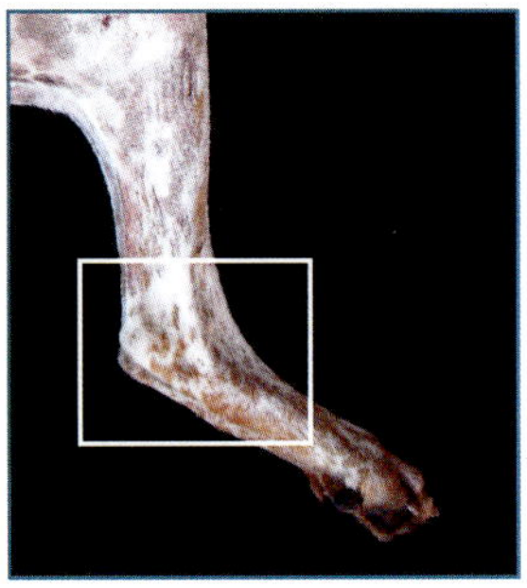

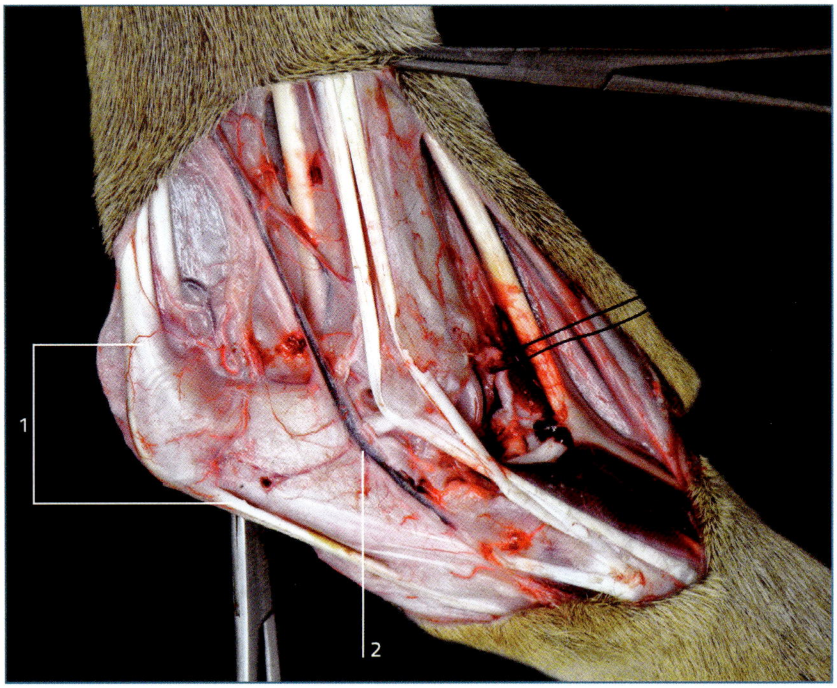

1 Superficial digital flexor muscle tendon
2 Lateral saphenous vein

2 At the tuber calcanei and the plantar edge the course of the superficial digital flexor tendon can be identified.

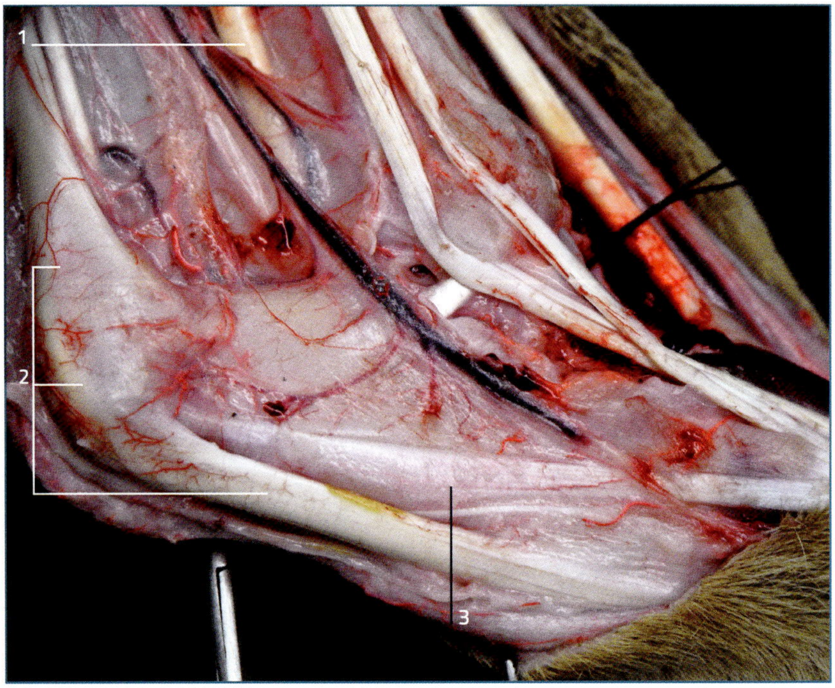

1 Deep digital flexor muscle tendon
2 Superficial digital flexor muscle tendon
3 Abductor muscle of the fifth toe

Approach to the calcaneus and the plantar region of the tarsal bones

1 This is continuation of the lateroplantar approach to the calcaneus as described above. The plantar region of the tarsus is exposed, incising the plantar fascia by sectioning the flexor retinaculum (dotted line) in order to access the plantar surface of the tarsus.

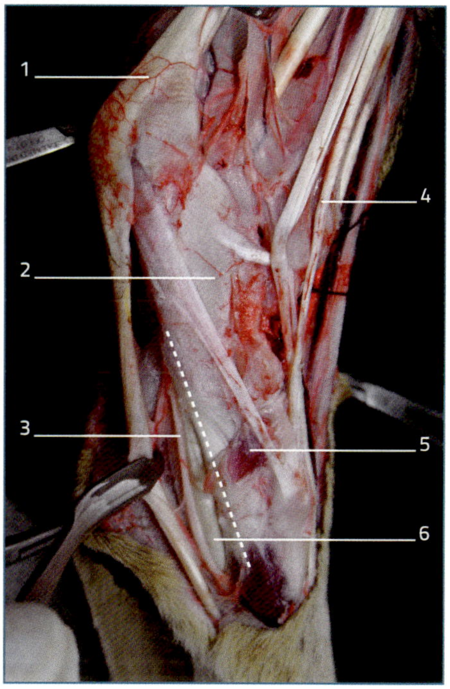

1 Superficial digital flexor muscle tendon
2 Body of calcaneus
3 Plantar nerves
4 Long fibular muscle tendon
5 Quadratus plantae muscle
6 Deep digital flexor muscle tendon

2 After sectioning the retinaculum, the deep digital flexor muscle is displaced towards the plantar area to allow plantar access to the calcaneus and the distal bones of the tarsus.

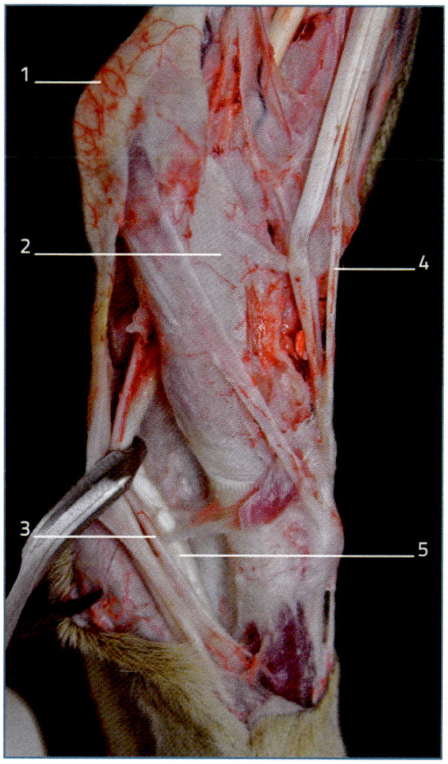

1 Superficial digital flexor muscle tendon
2 Body of calcaneus
3 Plantar nerves
4 Long fibular muscle tendon
5 Deep digital flexor muscle tendon

The images included for surgical approaches are adapted from: Latorre, R., Gil, F., Climent, S., López, O., Henry, R., Ayala, M., Ramírez, G., Martínez, F., Vázquez, J.M. *Color Atlas of Surgical Approaches to the Bones and Joints of the Dog and Cat*. Intermédica S.A., 2009; pp. 0-266. ISBN 978-950-555-353-2.

BIBLIOGRAPHY

Anatomy, diagnostic imaging techniques and surgical approaches

AGUINAGA, H.F., RIVERA, J.A., TAMAYO, L.J., TOBÓN, M., OSORNO, R.C. Tomografía axial computarizada y resonancia magnética para la elaboración de un atlas de anatomía segmentaria a partir de criosecciones axiales del perro. *Rev Col Cienc Pec*, 2006; Vol. 19:4.

CLIMENT, S. *et al. Manual de anatomía y embriología de los animales domésticos*. Conceptos básicos y datos aplicativos. Miembro torácico y miembro pelviano. Sistema circulatorio. Esqueleto de la cabeza. Ed. Acribia, 2004.

EVANS, H.E. *Miller's Anatomy of the Dog*, 3ª ed. WB Saunders, Philadelphia, 1993.

FRANCH, J., LÓPEZ, C. *Atlas de abordajes quirúrgicos en traumatología de pequeños animales*. Temis Pharma, S.L., 1999.

GARLAND, M.R., LAWLER, L.P., WHITAKER, B.R., WALKER, I.D., CORL, F.M., FISHMAN, E.K. Modern CT Applications in Veterinary Medicine. *RadioGraphics*, 2002; 22:55-62.

LATORRE, R., GIL, F., CLIMENT, S., LÓPEZ, O., HENRY, R., AYALA, M., RAMÍREZ, G., MARTÍNEZ, F., VÁZQUEZ, J.M. *Atlas en color sobre abordajes a huesos y articulaciones en el perro y en el gato*. Intermédica S.A., 2008; pp. 0-266. ISBN 978-950-555-347-1.

LATORRE, R., RAMÍREZ, G., LÓPEZ, O., ARENCIBIA, A., VÁZQUEZ, J.M., GIL, F., ORENES, M., MORENO, F. *Cuadernos prácticos de osteología veterinaria. Vol. III: Carnívoros.* Secretariado de Publicaciones e Intercambio Científico. Universidad de Murcia, 1995. ISBN 84-7684-650-9.

LUJÁN, A. Resonancia magnética (RM) y tomografía computerizada (TC) en patologías espinales seleccionadas. X Congreso de Especialidades Veterinarias de AVEPA. Valencia. Abril, 2011.

MONTEAGUDO, S., LISTE, F. Utilidad diagnóstica de la tomografía computerizada en la clínica veterinaria. *Consulta de difusión veterinaria*, 2010 Nov; 18(175):65-72.

Nómina anatómica veterinaria. 5th Editorial Committee Hannover, Columbia, Gent, Sapporo. 2005. International Committee on Veterinary Gross Anatomical Nomenclature World Association of Veterinary Anatomists (WAVA), 2005; pp. 1-190.

PIERMATTEI, D.L., JOHNSON, K.A. *An Atlas of Surgical Approaches to the Bones and Joints of the Dog and Cat*, 4th ed. Elsevier Inc, New York, 2006.

SANDOVAL, J. *Tratado de anatomía veterinaria*, 3ª ed. Tomo II: Aparato locomotor. Imprenta Sorles, León, 1998.

SCHALLER, O. *Nomenclatura anatómica veterinaria ilustrada*. Ed. Acribia, Zaragoza, 1992.

SOLER, M., MURCIANO, J., LATORRE, R., BELDA, E., AGUT, A. Ultrasonographic, computed tomographic and magnetic resonance imaging anatomy of the normal canine stifle joint. *The Veterinary Journal*, 2007; 174:351-361.

USÓN, J., SUN, F., CRISÓSTOMO, V., SÁNCHEZ, F.M., CLIMENT, S., LATORRE, R., MAYNAR, M. Manual de técnicas endoluminales y radiología intervencionista en veterinaria. Ed. Centro de Cirugía de Mínima Invasión Jesús Usón, 1ª Ed. Cáceres, 2010.

VILLAMONTE-CHEVALIER, A., SOLER, M., SARRIA, R., AGUT, A., LATORRE, R. Anatomical study of fibrous structures of the medial aspect of the canine elbow joint. *Veterinary Record*, 2012; 171(23):596 DOI: 10.1136/vr.100981.

WEISSE, C.W., BERENT, A.C., TODD, K.L., SOLOMON, J.A. Potential applications of interventional radiology in veterinary medicine. *J American Veterinary Medical Association*. November 15, 2008; Vol. 233, No. 10, pp. 1564-1574.

Orthopaedic conditions of the stifle joint

AIKEN, S.W. KASS, P.H., TOOMBS, J.P. Intercondylar notch width in dogs with and without cranial cruciate ligament injuries. *Vet Comp Orthop Traumatol*, 1995; 8:128-132.

ARAGON, C.L., BUDSBERG, S.C. Applications of evidence-based medicine: Cranial cruciate ligament injury repair in the dog. *Vet Surg*, 2005; 34:93-98.

ARNOCZKY, S.P. Surgery of the stifle. The cruciate ligaments (Part I). *Comp Cont Educ*, 1980; 11:106.

ARNOCZKY, S.P., TARVIN, G.B., MARSHALL, J.L. *et al*. Over-the-top procedure. Technique for anterior cruciate ligament substitution in the dog. *J Am Anim Hosp Assoc*, 1979; 15:283-290.

ARON, D.N., SELCER, B.A., SMITH, J.D. Autogenous tensor fascia lata graft replacement of the patellar ligament in a dog. *Vet comp Orthop Traumatol*, 1997; 10:141-145.

BANWELL, M.N., HOSGOOD, G., KERWIN, S.C. *et al*. In vitro evaluation of fluorocarbon leader line for use as a fabella-tibial suture. *Vet Comp Orthop Traumatol*, 2004; 17:35-40.

BAR-AM, Y., KLEMENT, E., FOURMAN, V. *et al*. Mechanical evaluation of two loop-fastening methods for stainless steel wire. *Vet Comp Orthop Traumatol*, 2004; 17:241-246.

BENNETT, D., CAMPBELL, J.R. Unusual soft tissue orthopaedic problems in the dog. *J Small Anim Prat*, 1979; 20:27-39.

BONNEAU, N.H., BRETON, L. Avulsion fracture of the origin of the extensor digitorum longus muscle in two Great Dane dogs. *J Vet Orthop*, 1984; 3:15-20.

BRINKER, W.O., OLMSTEAD, M.L., SUMNER-SMITH, G., PRIEUR, W.D. *Manual of internal fixation in small animals,* second revised edition. Springer, 1998.

BRUNNBERG, L., DÜRR, E., KNOSPE, C. Zu den verletzungen del Patella und Ligamentum patellae bei Hund und Katze I. Patellafraktur. *Kleintierpraxis*, 1991; 36:547-559.

BRUNNBERG, L., DÜRR, E., KNOSPE, C. Zu den verletzungen del Patella und Ligamentum patellae bei Hund und Katze II. Ruptur des Ligamentum patellae. *Kleintierpraxis*, 1992; 37:179-182.

CHAUVET, A.E., JOHNSON, A.L., PIJANOWSKI, G.J. *et al*. Evaluation of fibular head transposition, lateral fabellar suture, and conservative treatment of cranial cruciate ligament rupture in large dogs: a retrospective study. *J Am Anim Hosp Assoc*, 1996; 32:247- 255.

CHRISTOPHER, S.A., BEETEM, J., COOK, J.L. Comparison of long-term outcomes associated with three surgical techniques for treatment of cranial cruciate ligament disease in dogs. Vet Surg, 2013; 42:329-334.

DAMUR, D., TEPIC, S., MONTAVON, P.M. Proximal tibial osteotomy for the repair of cranial cruciate-deficient stifle joints in dogs. *Vet Comp Orthop Traumatol*, 2003; 4:211-216.

DE ROOSTER, H., DE BRUIN, T., VAN BREE, H. Morphologic and functional features of the canine cruciate ligaments. *Vet Surg*, 2006; 35:769-780.

DENNLER, R., KIPFER, N.M., TEPIC, S. *et al*. Inclination of the patellar ligament in relation to flexion angle in stifle joints of dogs without degenerative joint disease. *Am J Vet Res*, 2006; 67:1849-1854.

DICKINSON, C.R., NUNAMAKER, D.M. Repair of ruptured anterior cruciate ligament in the dog: experience of 101 cases, using a modified fascia strip technique. *J Am Vet Med Assoc*, 1977; 170:827-830.

DRAPE, J., GHITALLA, S., AUTEFAGE, A. Lésions méniscales et rupture du ligament croisé antérieur: étude rétrospective de 400 cas. *Le Point Vétérinaire*, 1990; 22:39-45.

DRAPE, J., GHITALLA, S., AUTEFAGE, A. Rupture du ligament croisé antérieur (LCA) chez le chien: pathologie traumatique ou dégénérative. *Le Point Vétérinaire*, 1990; 22:57-64.

DRAPE, J., GHITALLA, S., AUTEFAGE, A. Traitement chirurgical de la rupture du ligament croisé antérieur (LCA) chez le chien par la méthode “over the top” modifiée. *Le Point Vétérinaire*, 1990; 22:11-19.

DUVAL, J.M., BUDSBERG, S.C., FLO, G.L. *et al*. Breed, sex, and body weight as risk factors for rupture of the cranial cruciate ligament in young dogs. *J Am Vet Med Assoc*, 1999; 215:811-814.

ENDRES, B. Luxatio patellae congenita des Hundes. *Vet Med Diss*, München, 1977.

ENGELKE, A., MEYER-LINDENBERG, A., NOLTE, I. Die Ultraschalluntersuchung des inneren Kniegelenkes bei Hunden mit Kreuzbandriss. *Dtsch Tierärztl Wschr*, 1997; 104:114-117.

FRITZ, R.M. Zur Luxatio patellar des Hundes, klinisches und röntgenologisches Spätergebnis nach. Transposition der tuberositas tibiae und/oder vertiefung der Trochlea Ossis Femoris. *Vet Med Diss*, München, 1989.

GEYER, H. Die Behandlung der Kreuzbandrisse beim Hund: Vergleichende Untersuchungen. Vetsuisse Faculty, University of Zurich, Zurich, Switzerland, 1966.

GUERRERO, T., MAKARA, M., KATIOFSKY, K. *et al*. Comparison of healing of the osteotomy gap after tibial tuberosity advancement with and without the use of autogenous cancellous bone graft. Proceedings, 36th Annual Conference Veterinary Orthopedic Society, Steamboat Springs, Colorado, USA, 2009.

GUERRERO, T., MONTAVON, P.M. Advancement of the tibial tuberosity of cranial cruciate-deficient canine stifle. Video production: University of Zurich, 2003.

HAGEN, B. Untersuchungen zur apophysenfugenlösung und anderen Ossinfikationsstö-rungen im berich der tuberositas tibiae beim wachsenden Bullterrier. *Vet Med Diss*, München, 1991.

HAYASHI, K., MANLEY, P.A., MUIR, P. Cranial cruciate ligament pathophysiology in dogs with cruciate disease: A review. *J Am Anim Hosp Assoc*, 2004; 40:385-390.

HENDERSON, R.A, MILTON, J.L. The tibial compression mechanism: a diagnostic aid in stifle injuries. *J Am Anim Hosp Assoc*, 1978; 14:474-479.

HOFFMANN, D.E., MILLER, J.M., OBER, C.P. *et al*. Tibial tuberosity advancement in 65 canine stifles. *Vet Comp Orthop Traumatol*, 2006; 19:219-227.

HULSE, D.A., SHIRES, P., ABDELBAKI, Y.Z., HUGH-JONES, M., KEARNEY, M.T. Vascular access channeling to increase meniscal regeneration in the dog. *Vet Surg*, 1986; 15:414-419.

JAGER, M., WIRTH, C.J. *Praxis der Orthopädie*. Georg Thieme Verlag, 1986.

JERRAM, R.M., WALKER, A.M., WARMAN, C.G. Proximal tibial intraarticular ostectomy for treatment of canine cranial cruciate ligament injury. *Vet Surg*, 2005; 34:196-205.

KIM, S.E., POZZI, A., KOWALESKI, M.P. *et al*. Tibial osteotomies for cranial cruciate ligament insufficiency in dogs. *Vet Surg*, 2008; 37:111-125.

KIPFER, N.M., TEPIC, S., DAMUR, D.M. *et al*. Effect of tibial tuberosity advancement on femorotibial shear in cranial cruciate-deficient stifles. An in vitro study. *Vet Comp Orthop Traumatol*, 2008; 21:385-390.

KOESTLIN, R. Cirugía articular. I Congreso Internacional de la SETOV, Proceeding textbook 90, Cáceres, 2009.

KORVICK, D.L., JOHNSON, A.L., SCHAEFFER, D.J. Surgeons' preferences in treating cranial cruciate ligament ruptures in dogs. *J Am Vet Med Assoc*, 1994; 205:1318.

LAFAVER, S., MILLER, N.A., STUBBS, W.P. *et al*. Tibial tuberosity advancement for stabilization of the canine cranial cruciate ligament-deficient stifle joint: surgical technique, early results, and complications in 101 dogs. *Vet Surg*, 2007; 36:573-586.

LAMPMAN, T.J., LUND, E.M., LIPOWITZ, A.J. Cranial cruciate disease: current status of diagnosis, surgery, and risk for disease. *Vet Comp Orthop Traumatol*, 2003; 16:122-126.

MATIS, U. Zur Drahtzuggurtung distañer epiphysiolysen bzw. Suprakondylärer Frakturen des femurs bei Katze und Hund. *Bert Münch Tierärztl Wschr*, 1977; 90:240-243.

MATIS, U., KÖSTLIN, R. Zur Kreuzbandruptur bei der Katze. *Prak Teirarzt*, 1978; 59:585.

MOORES, A.P., BECK, A.L., JESPERS, K.J.M. *et al*. Mechanical evaluation of two crimp clamp systems for extracapsular stabilization of the cranial cruciate ligament-deficient canine stifle. *Vet Surg*, 2006; 35:470-475.

MULLEN, H.S., MATTHIESEN, D.T. Complications of transposition of the fibular head for stabilisation of the cranial cruciate-deficient stifle in dog: 80 cases (1982-1986). *J Am Vet Med Assoc,* 1989; 195:1267-1271.

NEWTON C.D., NUNAMAKER, D.M. *Textbook of small animal orthopaedics*. JB Lippincott Company, Philadelphia, 1985.

NISELL, R. Mechanics of the knee. A study of joint and muscle load with clinical applications. *Acta Orthop Scand*, 1985; Suppl 216:1-42.

Patterson, R.H., Smith, G.K., Gregor, T.P., Newton, C.D. Biomechanical stability of four cranial cruciate ligament repair techniques in the dog. *Vet Surg*, 1991; 20:85-90.

Piermattei, D.L., Flo, G.L. *Handbook of small animal orthopedics and fracture treatment*, third edition. WB Saunders Company, Philadelphia, 1997.

Pond, M.J. Avulsion of the extensor digitorum longus muscle in the dog: A report of four cases. *J Small Anim Pract*, 1973; 14:785-796.

Pozzi, A. *et al*. Pressure distributions on the medial tibial plateau after medial meniscal surgery and tibial plateau leveling osteotomy in dogs. *VCOT*, 2008; 21:8-14.

Read, R.A., Robins, G.M. Deformity of the proximal tibia in dogs. *Vet Rec*, 1982; 111:295-298.

Reif, U., Probst, C.W. Comparison of tibial plateau angles in normal and cranial cruciate deficient stifles of Labrador retrievers. *Vet Surg*, 2003; 32:385-389.

Salter, R.B., Harris, W.R. Injuries involving the epiphyseal plate. *Journal of Bone & Joint Surg*, 1963; 45-A:587.

Schäfer, H.-J. Vergleichende Untersuchung zur chirurgischen Behandlung des vorderen Kreuzbandrissies beim Hund mit der "modifizierten Over-the-Top" und der "Fibulakopfversetzungstechnik". *Vet Med Diss*, Hannover, 1991.

Schäfer, H.-J., Köstlin, R.G., Nolte, I. Zwei Methoden für die Kreuzban-operation im vergleich: Die Over-the-Top und die fibulakopfversetzungstechnik. *Kleintierpraxis*, 1991; 36:683.

Schebitz, H., Brass, W. (Hrsg): *Operationen an Hund und Katze*. Verlag Paul Parey, 1985.

Schmökel, H.G., Montavon, P.M. Versetzung der tuberositas tibiae mit einer Kranialisation bei der Patellaluxation beim Hund. *Kleintierpraxis*, 1993; 38:805-808.

Schwandt, C.S., Bohorquez-Vanelli, A., Tepic, S. *et al*. Angle between the patellar ligament and tibial plateau in dogs with partial rupture of the cranial cruciate ligament. *Am J Vet Res*, 2006; 67:1855-1860.

Selmi, A.L., Padilha, J.G. Rupture of the cranial cruciate ligament associated with deformity of the proximal tibia in five dogs. *J Small Anim Pract*, 2001; 42(8):390-393.

Singleton, W.B. The surgical correction of the stifle deformities in the dog. *J small Anim Pract*, 1969; 10:59-69.

Slocum, B. Cranial tibial wedge osteotomy: a technique for eliminating cranial tibial thrust in cranial cruciate ligament repair. *JAVMA*, 1984; 184:564-569.

Slocum, B., Devine, T. Cranial tibial wedge osteotomy: a technique for eliminating cranial tibial thrust in cranial cruciate ligament repair. *J Am Vet Med Assoc*, 1984; 184:564-569.

Slocum, B., Devine, T. Trochlear recession for correction of luxating patella in the dog. *J Am Vet Med Assoc*, 1985; 186(4):365-369.

Slocum, B., Slocum, D.B., Devine T., Boone, E. Wedge recession for treatment of recurrent luxation of the patella, A. preliminary report. *Clin Orthop Relat Res*, 1982; 164:48-53.

Slocum, B., Slocum, T.D. Tibial plateau leveling osteotomy for repair of cranial cruciate ligament rupture in the canine. *Vet Clin North Am Small Anim Pract*, 1993; 23(4):777-795.

Smith, G.K., Torg, J.S. Fibular head transposition for repair of cruciate-deficient stifle in the dog. *J Am Vet Med Assoc*, 1985; 187:375-383.

Stone, E.A., Betts, C.W., Rudy, R.L. Folding of the caudal horn of the medial meniscus secondary to severence of the cranial cruciate ligament. *Vet Surg*, 1980; 9:121-124.

Tepic, S., Damur, D., Montavon, P.M. Biomechanics of the stifle joint, Proceedings, 1st World Orthopedic Veterinary Congress ESVOT-VOS, Munich, 2002.

Vasseur, P.B. Stifle joint. In Slatter, D. (ed): *Textbook of Small Animal Surgery*, 3rd edition, vol. 2. Philadelphia, Saunders, 2003; pp. 2090-2116.

Vasseur, P.B., Johnson, A.L., Budsberg, S.C. *et al*. Randomized, controlled trial of the efficacy of craprofen, a nonsteroidal anti-inflammatory drug, in the treatment of ostearthritis in dogs. *J Am Vet Med Assoc*, 1995; 206:807-811.

Vasseur, P.B., Pool, R.R., Arnoczky, S.P. *et al*. Correlative biomechanical and histologic study of the cranial cruciate ligament in dogs. *Am J Vet Res*, 1985; 46:1842-1854.

VENZIN, C., HOWARD, J., RYTZ, U. *et al.* Tibial plateau angles with and without cranial cruciate ligament rupture - comparison between different dog populations and a wolf population. *Vet Comp Orthop Traumatol*, 2004; 17:232-236.

VÉREZ-FRAGUELA, J.L. Reparación de la rotura del ligamento cruzado anterior mediante osteotomía niveladora de la meseta tibial. *Consulta de Difus Vet*, 2001; 83 (9):77-90.

VOLLMERHAUS, B., SCHEBITZ, H., ROOS, H. Über die Entwicklung der Insertio ligamenti patellae beim wachsenden Hund. *Berl Münch Tierärztl Wschr*, 1981; 94:255-259.

VOSS, K., DAMUR, D.M., GUERRERO, T. *et al.* Force plate gait analysis to assess limb function after tibial tuberosity advancement in dogs with cranial cruciate ligament disease. *Vet Comp Orthop Traumatol*, 2008; 21:243-249.

WARZEE, C.C., DEJARDIN, L.M., ARNOCZKY, S.P., PERRY, R.L. Effect of tibial plateau leveling on cranial and caudal tibial thrusts in canine cranial cruciate-deficient stifles: an in vitro experimental study. *Vet Surg*, 2001; 30:278-286.

WESTHUES, M. Die Operation bei Zerreibug der Ligamenta decussata im Kniegelenk des Hundes und der Katze. In: Berge, E., Westhues, M. *Tierärztlichen Operationslehre*. 29 Auflage, S 365, Paul Parey verlag, 1969.

WHITEHAIR, J.G., VASSEUR, P.B., WILLITS, N.H. Epidemiology of cranial cruciate ligament rupture in dogs. *J Am Vet Med Assoc*, 1993; 203:1016-1019.

WILKE, V.L., CONZEMIUS, M.G., BESANCON, M.E. *et al.* Comparison of tibial plateau angle between clinically normal Greyhounds and Labrador Retrievers with and without rupture of the cranial cruciate ligament. *J Am Vet Med Assoc*, 2002; 221:1426-1429.

ZAERA, J.P. Comparación de la técnica en cuña y la trocleoplastia con y sin ácido hialurónico en el tratamiento de la luxación rotuliana en el perro; estudio experimental. Tesis Doctoral, Universidad Complutense de Madrid, 1993.

ZAHM, H. Die Ligamenta decussata im gesunden und arthrotischen Kniegelenk des Hundes. *Vet Med Diss*, München, 1964.

ZELTZMAN, P.A., PARE, B., JOHNSON, G.M. *et al.* Relationship between age and tibial plateau angle in dogs with cranial cruciate rupture. *J Am Anim Hosp Assoc*, 2005; 41:117-120.

Orthopaedic conditions of the hip joint

BARDET, J.F., LETOURNEL, E. Prothèse totale de la hanche chez le chien. *Prat Med Chir Anim Comp*, 1995; 30:555.

BRINKER, W.O., PIERMATTEI, D.L., FLO, G.L. Artrothesis. In: *Handbook of Small Animal Orthopaedics and Fracture Treatment*. Philadelphia, WB Saunders, 1990, p. 481.

DEJARDIN, L.M., PERRY, R.L. *et al.* The effect of triple pelvic osteotomy on hip force in dysplastic dogs: a theoretical analysis. *Vet Surg*, 1995; 25:14-120.

DUHATOIS, B. La triple ostéotomie pelvienne: étude rétrospective sur 173 cas. *Prat Méd Chir anim Comp*, 1997; 32.

GRAEHLER, R.A., WEIGLE, J.P. The effect of plate type, angle of ilial osteotomy, and degree of axial rotation on the structural anatomy of the pelvis. *Vet Surg*, 1994; 23:13-20.

HAUPTMAN, J., PRIEUR, W.D. The angle of inclination of the canine femoral head and neck. *Vet Surg*, 1979; 8:74.

KOCH, D.A., HAZEWINKEL, H.A.W. Radiographic evaluation and comparison of plate fixation after triple pelvic osteotomy in 32 dogs with hip dysplasia. *Vet Comp Orthop Trauma*, 1993; 6:9-16.

MEIJ, B. Experiences at the Small Animal of the Utrecht University. Triple Pelvic Osteotomy Wet Lab. ES-VOT Congress, 1998.

SCHRADER, S.C. Triple osteotomy of the pelvis and trochanteric osteotomy as a treatment for hip dysplasia in the immature dog: the surgical technique and results of 77 consecutive operatios. *J Am Vet Med Assoc*, 1986; 189:659-665.

SLOCUM, B., DEVINE, T. Dorsal acetabular rim radiographic view for evaluatrion of the canine hip. *J Am Anim Hosp Assoc*, 1990; 26:289-296.

SLOCUM, B., DEVINE, T. Pelvic osteotomy for axial rotation of the acetabular segment in dogs with hip dysplasia. *Vet Clin North Am Small Anim Pract*, 1992; 22:645-682.

SLOCUM, B., DEVINE, T. Pelvic osteotomy in the dog as treatment for hip dysplasia. *Sem Vet Med Surg*, 1987; 2:107-116.

SLOCUM, B., DEVINE, T. Pelvic osteotomy technique for axial rotation of the acetabular segment in dogs. *J Am Anim Hosp Assoc*, 1986; 22: 331-338.

SMITH, G.K., POPOVICH, C.A. Evaluation of risk factors for degenerative joint disease associated with hip dysplasia in dogs. *J Am Vet Med Assoc*, 1995; 206:642-647.

SUKHIANI, H.R., HOLMBERG, D.L. Pelvic canal narrowing caused by triple osteotomy in the dog. *Vet Comp Orthop Trauma*, 1994; 7:110-116.

VÉREZ-FRAGUELA J.L. Displasia de cadera en el perro. *Revista del Club Español del Schnauzer*, 1996; 1(6):22-25.

VÉREZ-FRAGUELA, J.L. Fracturas pélvicas y acetabulares en el perro. *Consulta de Difusión Veterinaria*, 1998; (6) 55:13-23.

VÉREZ-FRAGUELA, J.L. Triple osteotomía pélvica, planificación y selección de los casos, técnica quirúrgica, experiencia clínica de 98 casos. *Condroprotección vet*, 2000; 5:5-9.

Orthopaedic conditions of the elbow joint

AUTEFAGE, A., ASIMUS, E., MATHON, D. Les troubles de croissance de l´avant-bras chez le chien: conséquences sur l´articulation du coude. *Revue Med Ve*, 1993; 144:12 953-65.

BARDET, J.F. Arthroscopy of the elbow in dogs. Part I: The normal arthroscopy anatomy using the craniolateral portal. *VCOT*, 1997; 10:1-5.

BARDET, J.F. Arthroscopy of the elbow in dogs. Part II: The cranial portals in the diagnosis and treatment of the lesions of the coronoid process. *VCOT*, 1997; 10:60-6.

BEDFORD, P.G. BSAVA News. Control of hereditary elbow disease in pedigree dogs. *Journal Small Animal Practice*, 1994; 35(2):119-22.

BENNETT, D., DUFF, S.R., KENE, R.O., LEE, R. Osteochondritis dissecans and fragmentation of the coronoid process in the elbow joint of the dog. *Veterinary Record*, 1981: 109:329-36.

BOCCIA, F., ORTEGA, C. *Estudio semiológico del miembro anterior del perro. Su aplicación en el diagnóstico de enfermedades ortopédicas*. San Marcos, 1991; 59-70.

BOUCK, G.R., MILLER, C.W., TAVES, L. A comparison of surgical and medical treatment of fragmented coronoid process and osteochondritis dissecans of the canine elbow. *VCOT*, 1995; 8:177-83.

CARPENTER, L.G., SCHWARZ, P.D., LOWRY, J.E., PARK, D.R., STEIN, D.F. Comparison of radiologic imaging techniques for diagnosis of fragmented medial coronoid process of the cubital joint in dogs. *JAVMA*, 1993; 203:178-83.

CORLEY, E.A. Elbow dysplasia in the German Shephed dog. Dissertation Colorado State University. Fort Collins. Co., 1966.

CROSS, A.R., CHAMBERS, J.N. Ununited anconeal process of the canine elbow. *Continuing Education*, 1997; 3:349-360.

DURANTE, E.J., BRUSHA, H.C. Displasia de codo, *Analecta veterinaria*, 1998; 18-59.

FOX, S.M., BURBIDGE, H.M., BRAY, J.C., GUERIN, S.R. Ununited anconeal process: lag-screw fixation. *JAAHA*, 1996; vol 32:52-6.

HENRY JR, W.B. Radiographic diagnosis and surgical management of fragmented medial coronoid process in dogs. *JAVMA*, 1984; 184:799-805.

HUIBREGTSE, B.A., JOHNSON, A.L., MUHLBAUER, M.C., PIJANOWSKI, G.J. The effect of treatment of fragmented coronoid process on the development of osteoarthritis of the elbow. *JAAHA*, 1994; 30:190-5.

IWEG Abstracts of the 7 th annual meeting of the international elbow working group, Constance, Germany VCOT, 1996; 9:58-71.

KÖSTLIN, R. Cirugía articular del codo. IV Curso cirugía articular. Proceeding 19-25, 2005.

Langley-Hobbs, S.J., Carmichael, S. Management of a caudolateral radial head luxation in a five-month old shih tzu. *VCOT*, 1996; 9:186-9.

Lewis, D.D., Parker, R.B., Hager, D.A. Fragmented medial coronoid process of the canine elbow. *Continuing Education*, 1989; 11(3):703-14.

Ljunggren, G., Cawley, A.J., Archibald, J. Elbow dysplasia in the dog. *JAVMA*, 1966; 148:887-91.

Macpherson, G.C., Lewis, D.D., Johnson, K.A., Allen, G.S., Yovich, J.C. Fragmented coronoid process associated with premature distal radial physeal closure in four dogs. *VCOT*, 1992; 5:93-9.

Miyabayashi, T., Takyguchi, M., Schrader, S.C., Biller, D.S. Radiographic anatomy of the medial coronoid process of dogs. *JAAHA*, 1995; 31:125-32.

Padgett, G.A., Mostosky, U.V., Probst, C.W., Thomas, M.W., Krecke, C.F. The inheritance of osteochondritis dissecans and fragmented coronoid process of the elbow joint in Labrador Retrievers. *JAAHA*, 1995; 31:327-30.

Read, R.A., Armstrong, S.J., Black, A.P., Macpherson, G.C., Syovich, J.C., Davey, T. Relationship between physical signs of elbow dysplasia and radiographic score in growing Rottweilers. *JAVMA*, 1996; 209(8):1427-30.

Roy, R.G., Wallace, L., Johnston, G. A retrospective long-term evaluation of ununited anconeal process excision on the canine elbow. *Vet Comp Orthop Traumatol*, 1994; 7:94-97.

Sjöström, L., Kasström, H., Källberg, M. Ununited anconeal process in the dog. Pathogenesis and treatment by osteotomy of the ulna. *VCOT*, 1995; 8:170-6.

Slatter, D. *Textbook of small animal surgery*. 2° ed W.B. Saunders Co 1966-1980 Philadelphia, 1993.

Suess Jr, R.P., Trotter, E.J., Konieczynski, D., Todhunter, R.J., Bartel, D.L., Flanders, J.A. Exposure and postoperative stability of three medial surgical approaches to the canine elbow. *Veterinary Surgery*, 1994; 23:87-93.

Swenson, L., Audel, L., Hedhammar, A. Prevalence and inheritance of and selection for elbow artrosis in Bernese Mountain dogs and Rottweiler in Sweden and benefit: cost analysis of a screening and control program. *JAVMA*, 1997; 210(2):215-21.

Tobias, T.A., Miyabayashi, T., Olmstead, M.L., Edrick, L.A. Surgical removal of fragmented medial coronoid process in the dog: Comparative effects of surgical approach and age at time of surgery. *JAAHA*, 1994; 30:360-8.

Van Sickle, D. The relationship of ossification to canine elbow dysplasia. *J Am Anim Hosp Assoc*, 1966; 2:24-31.

Vérez-Fraguela, J.L. Húmero distal. V curso osteosintesis SETOV. Proceeding 29, 2006.

Vérez-Fraguela, J.L. La osteoartritis, el cartílago y su farmacología. Fármacos antiosteoartríticos de acción lenta que modifican la enfermedad. *Condroprotección vet*, 2001; 5:4-15.

Walde, I., Tellhelm, B. Fragmented medialcoronoid process of the ulna (FCP) and osteochondritis dissecans (OCD) of the canine elbow and hock joint. A review of literature, diagnosis and therapy. *Wiener Tierärztliche Monastsschrift*, 1991; 78:414-21.

Weinstein, M.J., Mongil, C.M., Smith, G.K. Orthopedic conditions of the Rottweiler-Part I. *Continuing Education*, 1995; 17(6):813-28.

Wind, A.P. Elbow incongruity and developmental elbow diseases in the dog: part I; part II. *J Am Anim Hosp Assoc*, 1986; 22:711-30.

Orthopaedic conditions of the shoulder joint

Berry, C.R. Evaluation of the canine elbow for fragmented medial coronoid process. *Vet Radiol & Ultrasound*, 1992; 33:273.

Bouck, G.R., Miller, C.W., Taves, C.L. A comparison of surgical and medical treatment of fragmented coronoid process and ostechondritis dissecans of the canine elbow. *VCOT*, 1995; 8:177.

Boulay, J.P. Fragmented medial coronoid process of the ulna in the dog. *Vet Clin Noth Am SAP*, 1998; 28:51.

DENNY, H.R., GIBBS, C. The surgical treatment of osteochondritis dissecans and ununited coronoid process in the canine ellbow joint. *J Small Anim Pract*, 1980; 21:323.

FOX, S. *et al*. Developmental anomalies of the canine elbow. *VCOT*, 1983; 605:-615.

FOX, S. Prematur closure of distal radial and ulnar physes in the dog. Part I. Pathogenesis and Diagnosis. *Comp Cont Educ*, 1984; 6:128.

FOX, S. Premature closure of distal radial and ulnar physes in the dog. Part II: Treatment. *Comp Cont Educ*, 1984; 6:212.

GILSON, S.D., PIERMATTEI, D.L., SCHWARZ, P.D. Treatment of humeroulnar subluxation with a dynamic proximal ulnar osteotomy. *Vet Surg*, 1989; 18:114.

GRONDALEN, J., LINGAAS, F. Arthrosis in the elbow joint of young rapidly growing dogs: a genetic investigation. *J Small Anim Pract*, 1991; 32:460.

GUTHRIE, S. Use a radiographic scoring technique for the assessment of dogs with elbow osteochondrosis. *J Small Anim Pract*, 1989; 30:639.

HUIBREGTSE, B.A., JOHNSON, A.L., MUHLBAUER, M.C., PIJANOWSKI, G.J. The effect of treatment of fragmented coronoid process on the development of osteoarthritis of the elbow. *JAAHA*, 1994; 30:190.

KELLER, G.G. *et al*. Correlation of radiographic, necropsy and histologic findings in 8 dogs with elbow dysplasia. *Veterinary radiology & Ultrasound*, 1997; 38: 272.

KÖSTLIN, R. Cirugía articular del Hombro. V Curso cirugía articular. Proceeding 19-25, 2006.

KROTSCHEK, U., HULSE, D.A., BAHR, A., JERRAM, R.M. Ununited anconeal process: lag-screw fixation with proximal ulnar osteotomy. *VCOT*, 2000; 13:212.

MAY, C., BENNETT, D. Medial epicondylar spur associated with lameness in dogs. *J Small Anim Pract*, 1988; 29(12):797-803.

MILTON, J.L., MONTGOMERY, R.D. Congenital elbow dislocations. *Vet Clin North Am*, 1987; 17:873.

MIYABAYASHI, T., TAKIGUCHI, M., SCHRADER, S.C., BILLER, D.S. Radiographic anatomy of the medial coronoid process of dogs. *JAAHA*, 1995; 31:125.

MORGAN, J., WIND, A., DAVIDSON, A. Elbow displasia. *Hereditary Bone and Joint Diseases in the Dog*. Schluetersche, 1999; 41-94.

PADGETT, G.A., MOSTOSKY, U.V., PROBST, C.W., THOMAS, M.W., KRECKE, C.F. The inheritance of the osteochondritis dissecans and fragmented coronoid process of the elbow joint in Labrador Retrievers. *JAAHA*, 1985; 31:327.

READ, R.A., ARMSTRONG, S.J., O'KEEFE, J.D., EGER, C.E. Fragmentation of the medial coronoid process of the ulna in dogs: A study of 109 cases. *J Small Anim Pract*, 1990; 31:330.

REICHLE, J.K., PARK, R.D., BAHR, A.M. Computed tomographic findings of dogs with cubital joint lameness. *Vet Radiol & Ultrasound*, 2000; 41:125.

ROBBINS, G.M. Some aspects of the radiographical examination of the canine elbow joint. *J Small Anim Pract*, 1980; 21:417.

SJÖSTRÖM, L., KASSTRÖM, H., KÄLLBERG, M. Ununited anconeal process in the dog. Pathogenesis and treatment by osteotomy of the ulna. *VCOT*, 1995; 8:170-6.

STUDDERT, V.P., LAVELLE, R.B., BEILHARZ, R.G., MASON, T.A. Clinical features and hereditability of osteochondrosis of the elbow in labrador retrievers. *J Small Anim Pract*, 1991; 32:557.

SWENSON, L., AUDELL, L., HEDHAMMAR, A. Prevalence and inheritance of and selection for elbow arthrosis in Bernese Mountain dogs and Rottweilers in Sweden and benefit: cost analysis of a screening and control programm. *JAVMA*, 1997; 210(2):215-221.

WOSAR, M.A., LEWIS, D.D., NEUTWIRTH, L. *et al*. Radiographic evaluation of elbow joint before and after surgery in dogd with possible fragmented medial coronoid process. *J Am Vet Med Assoc*, 1999; 214:52.

ZONTINE, W.J. *et al*. Redifined type of elbow dysplasia involving calcified flexor tendons attached to the medial humeral epicondyle in three dogs. *JAVMA*, 1989; 194(8):1082-1085.

Orthopaedic conditions of the carpal and tarsal joints

DEE, J.F., DEE, J., PIERMATTEI, D.L. Classification, management, and repair of central tarsal fractures in the racing greyhound. *J Am Anim Hosp Assoc*, 1976; 12:398.

DOVERSPIKE, M., VASSEUR, P.B. Clinical findings and complications after talocrural artrodesis in dogs. *JAAHA*, 1991; 27:553.

EULENBURG, K. The use of the external fixator in ankle-joint injuries of dogs and cats. Therapy and results (1985-1995).Thesis, Munich, 1997.

FISCHER, H. Tarsal injuries in the cat. A review of 133 cases. Thesis, Munich, 1986.

GORSE, M.J., EARLY, T.D., ARON, D. Tarsocrural arthrodesis: Long-term functional results. *JAAHA*, 1991; 27:231.

GÖSSMANN, M. Tarsocrural injuries in the dog. A review of 142 cases. Thesis, Munich, 1984.

JOHNSON, S.G., HULSE, D.A., VANGUNDY, T.E., GREEN, R.W. Corrective osteotomy for pes varus in Dachshund. *Vet Surg*, 1989; 18:373.

KASA, G., KASA, F. Corrective osteotomy in case of the distal varus deviation of the tibia in dogs. *Kleintierpraxis*, 1982; 27:377.

KLAUSE, S.E., PIERMATTEI, D.L., SCHWARZ, P.D. Tarsocrural arthrodesis: Complications and recommendations. *VCOT*, 1989; 3:119.

MAUTERER, J.V., PRATA, R.G., CARBERRY, C.A., SCHRADER, S.C. Displacement of the tendon of the superficial digital flexor muscle in dogs: 10 cases (1983-1991). *J Am Vet Med Assoc*, 1993; 203:1162.

MAYRHOFER, E. Metaphyseal tibiadysplasia in Dachshounds. *Kleintierpraxis*, 1977; 22:223.

MÜLLER-ROHRMOSER, M. Carpal and tarsal arthrodesis in dogs and cats. Therapy and results (1985-1996). Thesis, Munich, 1997.

REINKE, J.D., MUGHANNAM, A.J., OWENS, J.M. Avulsion of the gastrocnemius tendon in 11 dogs. *J Am Anim Hosp Assoc*, 1993; 29:410.

REINKE, J.D., MUGHANNAM, A.J. Lateral luxation of the superficial digital flexor tendon in 12 dogs. *J Am Anim Hosp Assoc*, 1993; 29:303.

Published by Servet editorial - Grupo Asís Biomedia S.L.